W.W. Fleischhacker and D.J. Brooks (eds.)

Addiction
Mechanisms, Phenomenology and Treatment

SpringerWienNewYork

Prof. Dr. W. W. Fleischhacker
Department of Biological Psychiatry
Innsbruck University Clinics
Anichstrasse 35
A-6020 Innsbruck, Austria

Prof. Dr. D.J. Brooks
MRC Cyclotron Unit
Hammersmith Hospital
Du Cane Road
London W12 0NN, United Kingdom

Printed in Austria

Typesetting: Best-Set Typesetter Ltd., Hong Kong
Printing: A. Holzhausen's Nfg., A-1140 Wien

Printed on acid-free and chlorine-free bleached paper

SPIN: 10925195

CIP data applied for

With 9 (partly coloured) Figures

ISBN 3-211-01315-6 (hard cover) Springer-Verlag Wien New York
ISBN 3-211-01316-4 Journal of Neural Transmission [Suppl 66]
(soft cover) Springer-Verlag Wien New York

Preface

Addiction was the topic of the 6th Neuropsychiatry Symposium of the European Institute of Health Care. Substance related disorders rank among the leading causes for disability worldwide and represent a major concern in the field of public health. Ever since mankind has experienced the effects of psychotropic agents, first reports date back more than 5000 years, abuse and addiction have been a part of this story. Although the phenomenology and course of substance use disorders have long been known, especially since extensive research in the last century, neurobiological mechanisms behind these syndromes have only begun to unravel in the last few decades. The methodological progress in neuroimaging and molecular biology have significantly contributed to this process. The increasing knowledge about the way our brains' networks, with the dopaminergic inputs to the nucleus accumbens as one of the areas of key interest with regard to reward and reinforcement mechanisms, has led to a fascinating new look onto an old field. At this moment this field faces two major challenges: firstly to translate findings from preclinical, animal work to humans and secondly to develop treatment strategies based on this.

For the present volume, we have brought together experts, which cover a lot of this ground: consequently, the authors shed new light on the field from various different angles and discuss different drugs of abuse, ranging from the more traditional ones (like opiates and alcohol) to more recent additions, such as designer drugs. The treatment of addiction is also explored from different perspectives including pharmacological and psychotherapeutic approaches. On the threshold of a new area of addiction research, this volume is expected to wet the readers appetite to learn more about this exciting field of interdisciplinary research.

Innsbruck and London, July 2003

W. W. Fleischhacker
D. J. Brooks

Contents

The neurobiology of addiction

R. Maldonado

Laboratori de Neurofarmacologia, Facultat de Ciències de la Salut i de la Vida, Universitat Pompeu Fabra, Barcelona, Spain

Summary. Drug addiction includes complex neurobiological and behavioural processes. Acute reinforcing effects of drugs of abuse are responsible for the initiation of drug addiction, whereas the negative consequences of drug abstinence have a crucial motivational significance for relapse and maintenance of the addictive process. The mesocorticolimbic system represents a common neuronal substrate for the reinforcing properties of drugs of abuse. Both dopamine and opioid transmission play a crucial role in this reward pathway. Common neuronal changes have also been reported during the abstinence to different drugs of abuse that could underlie the negative motivational effects of withdrawal. These changes include decreased dopaminergic activity in the mesolimbic system and a recruitment of the brain stress pathways. All drugs of abuse interact with these brain circuits by acting on different molecular and neurochemical mechanisms. The existence of bidirectional interactions between different drugs of abuse, such as opioids and cannabinoids, provides further findings to support this common neurobiological substrate for drug addictive processes.

Introduction

Drug addiction has been defined as a behavioural pattern of drug use, characterized by overwhelming involvement with the use of a drug, the securing of its supply, and a high tendency to relapse after withdrawal (Jaffe, 1990). Addictive processes represent, hence, a chronic relapsing brain disorder characterized by neurobiological changes leading to compulsive drug seeking and taking despite adverse consequences or as loss control over drug use. All addictive drugs alter brain functioning and neurochemistry in a number of similar ways. Thus, biochemical, anatomical and electrophysiological studies have identified several neuroanatomical and neurochemical pathways that could represent a common substrate for the addictive properties of several drugs of abuse (Koob and LeMoal, 2001). Indeed, these systems include the brain stress circuits, and the dopamine and endogenous opioid systems which have many different projection sites and physiological functions. The central dopamine pathways have critical roles not only in the reward and motor systems but also in higher-order functions, such as cognition and memory (Grant et al., 1996). Opioid pathways within the central nervous system have been also involved in several essential functions, including pain and emotional processes (Van Ree et al., 1999).

Processes involved in drug addiction are complex from a neurobiological and behavioural point of view. Tolerance and physical dependence are adaptive responses to the prolonged exposure of neurons to different drugs, but only provide a partial correlate of their addictive properties. The main factor common to all drugs of abuse is their ability to induce drug-seeking behaviour, which is due to the positive reinforcing effects of the drugs. The relevance of the abstinence syndrome in drug compulsive use has been controversial (Jaffe, 1990; Koob and LeMoal, 1997), although increasing evidence suggests that the presence of a negative affective withdrawal state is important for maintenance of the addictive process (Koob and LeMoal, 1997).

Different models are available to evaluate tolerance and physical dependence in animals. The quantification of the withdrawal syndrome that appears after the disruption of a repeated drug administration permits the assessment of the severity of physical dependence. Tolerance is determined by evaluating the decreased pharmacological effects of a drug after repeated administration (Jaffe, 1990). However, during repeated drug administration a psychomotor sensitization, as defined by increased locomotor activation, can be also observed. Sensitization is mainly induced in animals by using an intermittent exposure schedule, and has been interpreted as a manifestation of the progressive increase in the incentive-salience state described as "wanting" that occurs after repeated exposure to drugs of abuse in humans (Robinson and Berridge, 1993). Several behavioural models have been used to evaluate the reinforcing effects of drugs of abuse. Indirect indices of reinforcement can be evaluated through the ability of a drug to module the reinforcing properties of other rewards (e.g. intracranial self-stimulation techniques) or to impart reinforcing properties on previously neutral stimuli or environments (e.g. place conditioning paradigm). Drug reinforcement can also be directly evaluated by using operant self-administration paradigms (Schulteis et al., 1997). The use of these experimental models in animal studies has provided information for understanding the behavioural and neurobiological mechanisms involved in the different components of drug addiction.

Processes involved in the initiation and maintenance of drug addiction

Koob and LeMoal (1997) have proposed that drug addiction processes progressively develop as a cycle of spiralling dysregulation of brain reward systems that continuously increases, resulting in compulsive drug use and a loss of control over drug-taking, which define the addictive state. The beginning of this addiction cycle starts with the first drug intake, and involves the development of an adaptive process that is initiated to counter the acute effects of the drug (Koob and LeMoal, 1997). Indeed, the organism maintains a homeostatic equilibrium in all of its system, including the brain reward system. The administration of a drug of abuse will challenge this homeostasis, and is therefore met with adaptive counter actions. In spite of these counteradaptive processes, that are part of a normal homeostatic limitation of reward function, neuronal circuits involved in reward fail to return within the normal physiological range (Koob et al., 1989). Thus, counteradaptations slowly develop in order to oppose the initial hedonic effects of a drug, they become larger over time and mask such initial hedonic effects (Solomon and Corbit, 1974). If these challenges persist, the organism must accomplish an enormous effort to modify different physiological parameters in order to maintain apparent stability. This system is at the limit of its capability and a small challenge can lead to breakdown. Such dysregulations grow with repeated drug intake producing a pathological state that drives further drug intake, which in turn exaggerates the pathological state (Koob and LeMoal, 2001).

These addictive processes have been linked both to the positive reinforcing properties of the drugs and to the effects of these drugs in terminating the negative consequences of the withdrawal syndrome. Acute reinforcing effects of drugs of abuse seem to be responsible for the initiation and establishment of drug addiction (Koob, 1992). However, the acute effects of initial drug intake triggers the beginning of counteradaptive mechanisms such as neuroadaptation within the dopamine and endogenous opioid systems and activation of brain stress circuits (Koob and LeMoal, 2001). Negative affective withdrawal state related to these counteradaptive changes may not only signal the beginning of the development of dependence, but may have a crucial motivational significance for relapse and maintenance of the addictive process (Koob and LeMoal, 1997).

Important advances have been recently obtained in the knowledge of the neurobiological substrate of both the reinforcing properties and the negative effects of the withdrawal syndrome to the different drugs of abuse. Those studies provide increasing evidence for the existence of multiple common neurochemical, neuroanatomical and molecular mechanisms to explain these complex processes.

Neurobiology of drug reinforcement

Experimental evidence indicates that the mesocorticolimbic dopaminergic system represents a common neuronal substrate for the motivational and rewarding properties of most of the drugs of abuse (Koob, 1992). The major components of this drug reward circuit are the ventral tegmental area, containing the dopaminergic cell bodies, and the terminal areas in the basal forebrain (nucleus accumbens, olfactory tubercle, amygdala, and frontal and limbic cortices) (Koob and LeMoal, 2001). Both dopamine and opioid transmission play a crucial role in this reward pathway. However, other neurotransmitter systems also interact with this reward circuit, such as GABA, glutamate and serotonin (Koob, 1992). Dopamine projections that modulate forebrain and cortical areas act in parallel with related sets of structures. Two of these complex of structures are particularly relevant for drug addictive processes: the mesolimbic-accumbens-amygdaloid complex, mainly the extended amygdala and nucleus accumbens shell (Alheid and Heimer, 1988; Koob, 1999), and the cortico-striatal-pallidal-thalamic-circuit, especially the frontal and cingulate cortices (Koob and LeMoal, 2001). The first set of structures is involved in drug acute reinforcing effects. Indeed, prototypical drugs of abuse, including opioids, psychostimulants, cannabinoids, alcohol and nicotine, increase the discharge rate of mesolimbic dopamine neurons (Matthews and German, 1984; Mereu et al., 1984, 1987; Chen et al., 1991; Pontieri et al., 1996; Gessa et al., 1998). In vivo microdialysis studies have revealed that such activation induced by acute administration of virtually all major drugs of abuse is associated with increased dopamine output in innervated projection structures, mainly in the shell of the nucleus accumbens (Di Chiara and Imperato, 1988; Pontieri et al., 1995, 1996; Tanda et al., 1997). Drug-seeking behaviour under the control of reinforcing processes that result from other conditioned stimuli may depend ultimately on the extended amygdala and involve cortical projections to the core of the nucleus accumbens which is anatomically related to the striatal-pallidal circuit (Everitt et al., 1999; Koob and LeMoal, 2001). The cortico-striatal-pallidal-thalamic-circuit is closely related to cognitive functioning and compulsive repetitive behaviours, and is activated during intense drug craving, as visualized by neuroimaging techniques (Volkow and Fowler, 2000).

All drugs of abuse interact with these brain circuits by different molecular and neurochemical mechanisms (Koob and LeMoal, 2001). Thus, opioids enhance the activity of the dopamine mesolimbic system by decreasing the activity of GABA neurons, which inhibit dopamine cells in the ventral tegmental area. Dopamine independent mechanisms within the nucleus accumbens also seem involved in opioid reinforcing effects (Pettit et al., 1984; Shippenberg et al., 1992; Spyraki et al., 1983). Psychostimulants directly enhance mesolimbic dopamine activity by blocking monoamine transporter proteins which results in a blockade of monoamine reuptake, and in some cases also produces an increase in monoamine release (Rudnick and Clark, 1993). Cannabinoids also enhance the dopamine mesolimbic activity (Chen et al., 1991), and high levels of CB1 cannabinoid receptors are present in the nucleus accumbens (Tsou et al., 1998). Thus, cannabinoids have been reported to decrease the activity of excitatory glutamatergic afferents to the nucleus accumbens that contact with the accumbens GABA interneurons (Robbe et al., 2001). Nicotinic acetylcholine receptors are also present in the mesolimbic system (Pontieri et al., 1996), and nicotine may increase dopamine activity and opioid peptide transmission in this mesolimbic circuitry (Corrigall et al., 1992). Cholinergic input to ventral tegmental area from the pedunculopontine tegmental nucleus could participate in these nicotine effects (Picciotto and Corrigall, 2002). Dopamine (Pfeffer and Samson, 1988) and opioid peptide (Heyser et al., 1999; Roberts et al., 2000) activity within the mesolimbic system also contribute to the reinforcing actions of ethanol. However, other neurotransmitters also participate in the rewarding effects of ethanol, including facilitation of $GABA_A$ activity, inhibition of NMDA glutamate receptors and interaction with several serotonergic receptors ($5HT_{1A}$, $5HT_2$ and $5HT_3$)

(Lovinger et al., 1989; Richards et al., 1991; Eckardt et al., 1998; Roberts et al., 1998).

Interestingly, the development of psychomotor sensitization to drugs of abuse is associated with a number of neurochemical changes within the mesolimbic dopamine system (White, 1996), which suggests the involvement of the same neurochemical and neuroanatomical pathways in both sensitization and the acute reinforcing effects of drugs (Koob and Bloom, 1988).

Neurobiology of drug withdrawal manifestations

Acute withdrawal from the chronic use of several drugs of abuse is associated with physical signs, with different manifestations depending on the drug. However, physical symptoms of withdrawal may have few relevance to the motivation to take drugs. Drug withdrawal is also associated with subjective symptoms of negative affect, such as dysphoria, depression, irritability and anxiety, and dysregulation of brain reward systems. These motivational changes associated with drug withdrawal have been postulated to be an important component for maintaining addiction, and involve some of the same neurochemical systems participating in the rewarding effects of drugs of abuse, such as the dopamine system (Koob and LeMoal, 2001). Indeed, an important common change occurring in the mesolimbic system during abstinence to different drugs of abuse (psychostimulants, opioids, cannabinoids, nicotine and ethanol) is a marked decreased of the dopaminergic activity. The spontaneous firing rate of ventral tegmental area dopamine neurons has been reported to be attenuated during abstinence to several drugs of abuse (Diana et al., 1993, 1998). In agreement, in vivo microdialysis studies have revealed a profound decrease in dopamine levels in the nucleus accumbens during opioid (Acquas et al., 1991; Acquas and Di Chiara, 1992; Rossetti et al., 1992), psychostimulants (Parsons et al., 1991; Rossetti et al., 1992), ethanol (Rossetti et al., 1992; Diana et al., 1993) and nicotine (Hilderbrand et al., 1998) withdrawal syndrome. This decreased dopaminergic activity seems to be related to the aversive/dysphoric consequences of cannabinoid withdrawal.

Another common change observed during the drug withdrawal syndrome is a recruitment of the brain stress circuitry. Thus, the withdrawal syndrome to several drugs of abuse such as opioids, psychostimulants, cannabinoids and ethanol, includes an important elevation in extracellular levels of corticotropin-releasing factor (CRF) in the mesolimbic system, mainly in the central nucleus of the amygdala (Cummings et al., 1983; Koob, 1996; Merlo-Pick et al., 1995; Rodriguez de Fonseca et al., 1997). This alteration of the limbic CRF function may have a motivational role in mediating the stress-like symptoms and negative affect that accompany drug withdrawal syndrome. CRF function in the pituitary adrenal is also activated during acute drug withdrawal and the dysregulation of the hypothalamic-pituitary axis may persist even after acute withdrawal (Kreek et al., 1984).

Compensatory changes in the intracellular signalling systems, mainly involving the cyclic AMP pathway, have been reported during the withdrawal syndrome to some drugs of abuse such as opioids and cannabinoids. These changes seem to play an important role in the somatic manifestations of the physical abstinence. Initially, acute activation of opioid (Sharma et al., 1975) and cannabinoid (Howlett and Fleming, 1984) receptors leads to an inhibition of adenylyl cyclase activity. In contrast, during opioid (Nestler and Tallman, 1988) and cannabinoid (Hutcheson et al., 1998) withdrawal adenylyl cyclase activity was increased in some specific brain structures. Similar increases were also observed during chronic opioid and/or cannabinoid treatment in other intracellular components of the cyclic AMP pathway, such as G protein levels (Nestler et al., 1989), cyclic AMP levels (Rubino et al., 2000a), cyclic AMP-dependent protein kinase activity (Nestler and Tallman, 1988; Rubino et al., 2000b), the phosphorylation state of the transcription factor CREB (Guitart et al., 1992) and a number of cyclic AMP-regulated phosphoproteins, including tyrosine hydroxylase, the rate-limiting enzyme in the biosynthesis of catecholamines (Guitart and Nestler, 1989). In spite of the involvement of this common intracellular pathway in cannabinoid and opioid dependence, different brain structures have been reported to participate in the physical manifestations of opioid and cannabinoid withdrawal. Thus, locus coeruleus and other brainstem structures, such as the periaqueductal gray matter, are responsible for the somatic signs of opioid withdrawal syndrome (Maldonado et al., 1992). In the case of cannabinoid dependence, the cerebellum seems to play a crucial role for the somatic expression of THC withdrawal (Hutcheson et al., 1998; Tzavara et al., 2000).

Long-term neural adaptive changes induced by drugs of abuse

Drugs of abuse produce long-term adaptive changes in the brain that may contribute to drug addiction and to the vulnerability to relapse even long time after the last drug intake. A first hypothesis for explaining these long-term changes is provided by the existence of similar molecular mechanisms involved in learning and memory processes, and drug addiction (Ungless et al., 2001). Indeed, both processes are modulated by the same neurochemical systems and share some intracellular signalling cascades. For instance, the molecular mechanism involved in the enhancement induced by cocaine in glutamatergic transmission in the ventral tegmental area seems to be similar to that associated with long-term potentiation in the hippocampus (Ungless et al., 2001), which is directly linked with memory and learning (Hyman and Malenka, 2001). In addition, the activation of the transcription factor CREB has been linked to both learning and memory (Bourtchuladze et al., 1994), and drug addiction processes (Maldonado et al., 1996). In spite of this common neurochemical mechanisms, different brain regions have been classically proposed to be involved in learning and memory processes, and drug addiction. Whereas hippocampus is crucial for learning and memory, the mesolimbic system represents the main substrate for drug reinforcing. However, there is also substantial convergence of the neural circuits involved in learning and memory, and drug addiction (Nestler, 2001). Thus, animals maintain electrical self-stimulation in the hippocampus, indicating the relevance of this region in rewarding responses (Wise, 1996). On the other hand, the nucleus accumbens modulates the emotional value and by this way controls the strength of memories encoded in the hippocampus (Nestler, 2001).

Repeated administration of drugs of abuse is also able to produce changes in neuronal gene expression, which represent one possible mechanism to explain the long-term behavioural and neural alterations that persist for long periods even in the absence of drug administration (Hyman and Nestler, 1996). Transcription factors, which bind to regulatory elements in the promoter of their target genes, play a major role in these long-term adaptive changes. Thus, acute and chronic administration of different drugs of abuse modify several proteins belonging to the transcription factor activator-protein-1 (AP-1), such as the Fos family members (Karin et al., 1997). Acute exposure to several drugs of abuse produces a rapid and transient induction of c-Fos and other Fos family members in the nucleus accumbens and striatum. In contrast, repeated exposure to these drugs induces isoforms of ΔFosB whereas the induction of c-Fos and other Fos-like proteins is then desensitized (Hope et al., 1994; Chen et al., 1995; Nye et al., 1995; Moratalla et al., 1996). In contrast to other proteins of the Fos family, isoforms of ΔFosB are extremely stable, and once induced, they remain detectable in the brain for weeks to months, even in the absence of further drug administration (Kelz and Nestler, 2000). Isoforms of ΔFosB are accumulated only after chronic, but not after acute drug administration. Many types of chronic stimuli are able to induce ΔFosB, but the induction occurs in different brain structures depending on the stimuli (Kelz and Nestler, 2000). A selective induction of ΔFosB in the nucleus accumbens and the striatum has been reported after repeated administration of several drugs of abuse, such as psychostimulants (Nye et al., 1995), opioids (Nye and Nestler, 1996), nicotine (Pich et al., 1997) and ethanol (Ryabinin and Wang, 1998). Interestingly, expression of ΔFosB has been shown to increase the sensitivity to hyperlocomotor and rewarding effects of psychostimulants in rats (Kelz et al., 1999). ΔFosB expression has been also reported to increase the sensitivity to opioid rewarding effects (Keltz and Nestler, 2000). Therefore, ΔFosB is an attractive candidate to serve as a molecular switch that mediates long-lasting adaptive changes induced in the brain by repeated administration of drugs of abuse (Kelz and Nestler, 2000).

Interactions between different drugs of abuse: bidirectional opioid/cannabinoid interactions

Additional findings to support the existence of common neurobiological pathways on drug addictive processes are provided by the bidirectional interactions between different drugs of abuse. The interactions that have been reported between opioid and cannabinoid dependence represent a clear example (Maldonado, 2003). Thus, the blockade of the endogenous cannabinoid system by the administration of a selective antagonist of the centrally located CB-1 cannabinoid receptors (SR 141716A) precipitated several behavioural and biochemical manifestations of opioid withdrawal in morphine-dependent animals (Navarro et al., 1998). Additionally, the opioid antagonist naloxone precipitated behavioural signs of cannabinoid withdrawal in rats chronically treated with cannabinoid agonists (Kaymakcalan et al., 1977; Navarro et al., 1998). Acute administration of THC (Hine et al., 1975a,b; Lichtman et al., 2001) or the endogenous cannabinoid anandamide (Vela et al., 1995) has been reported to attenuate the severity of naloxone-precipitated morphine withdrawal. A similar effect was observed when THC was administered for a long period of time before starting opioid dependence. Thus, chronic pretreatment with THC before starting chronic opioid administration, decreased the somatic manifestations of naloxone-precipitated morphine withdrawal and did not modify morphine rewarding effects (Valverde et al., 2001). Therefore, the long-term pre-exposure to cannabinoids does not seem to modify motivational responses of opioids that are related to their addictive properties.

Recent studies using knockout mice have clarified the involvement of the endogenous opioid system in the different components of cannabinoid abstinence (Maldonado and Rodriguez de Fonseca, 2002). Thus, the severity of SR 141716A-precipitated cannabinoid withdrawal was significantly decreased in THC dependent knockout mice lacking the pre-proenkephalin gene (Valverde et al., 2000), but was not modified in knockout mice deficient in the prodynorphin gene (Zimmer et al., 2001). The behavioural expression of cannabinoid withdrawal has also been evaluated in knockout mice lacking the different opioid receptors. THC withdrawal syndrome was not modified in single knockout mice deficient in delta or kappa opioid receptors (Ghozland et al., 2001). In single knockout mice deficient in mu opioid receptors, cannabinoid abstinence was not modified (Ghozland et al., 2001) or resulted decreased when using very high doses of THC (Lichtman et al., 2001). However, a dramatic attenuation in the severity of cannabinoid withdrawal was observed in double knockout mice lacking both mu and delta opioid receptors (Castañé et al., 2003). Therefore, a simultaneous activation of mu and delta opioid receptors, probably by endogenous opioid peptides derived from pre-proenkephalin is required for the somatic expression of cannabinoid abstinence. Interestingly, this interaction between cannabinoid and opioid dependence seems to be bidirectional. Indeed, a decrease in the severity of morphine withdrawal syndrome was also reported in knockout mice deficient in CB-1 cannabinoid receptors indicating that the endogenous cannabinoid system participates in the somatic expression of opioid abstinence (Ledent et al., 1999).

The involvement of the endogenous opioid system in the motivational effects of cannabinoids has been also investigated in knockout mice lacking mu, delta or kappa opioid receptors (Ghozland et al., 2002). THC-induced rewarding effects in the place conditioning paradigm were abolished in mu opioid receptor knockout mice, but were not modified in mice lacking delta or kappa opioid receptors. In agreement with these results, non-selective opioid antagonists (naloxone and naltrexone) attenuated self-administration behaviour induced by THC (Goldberg et al., 2001) and by the cannabinoid agonist CP 55,940 (Braida et al., 2001). On the other hand, the dysphoric effects induced by a high dose of THC were not modified in delta opioid receptor knockout mice, slightly attenuated in mu knockout animals and completely abolished in mice lacking kappa opioid receptor, suggesting a crucial role of kappa receptor in THC-induced dysphoria (Ghozland et al., 2002). Results obtained with knockout mice deficient in the prodynorphin gene are in agreement with this hypothesis. Thus, the conditioned place aversion induced by a high dose of THC was completely abolished in these prodynorphin knockout mice (Zimmer et al., 2001). Therefore, mu opioid receptors are crucial for the rewarding effects of cannabinoids whereas kappa opioid receptors, probably activated by opioid peptides derivative from prodynorphin, mediate the aversive responses induced by these drugs. This interaction between the cannabinoid and opioid systems on motivational responses also seems to be bidirectional. Indeed, the rewarding effects induced by morphine in the conditioned place preference paradigm (Martin et al., 2000) and morphine-induced intravenous self-administration (Ledent et al., 1999) were blocked in knockout mice deficient in CB-1 cannabinoid receptors. In agreement, blockade of CB-1 cannabinoid receptors by SR-141716A administration partially reversed heroin-induced intracerebroventricular self-administration (Braida et al., 2001).

Concluding remarks

Drug addiction includes complex neurobiological and behavioural processes, where both the positive reinforcing properties of the drug and the negative effects related to drug abstinence play a decisive role. Recent findings support the multiplicity of studies suggesting the existence of common neurobiological mechanisms for both the reinforcing effects and the negative withdrawal consequences of most drugs of abuse. This information is based on anatomical, biochemical and molecular studies showing the crucial role played by the mesolimbic dopaminergic pathways, the endogenous opioid system, and the brain and pituitary stress systems in these addictive processes. Drugs of abuse interact with these common brain circuits producing neuroadaptations and counteradaptive changes leading to a profound dysregulation of brain motivational and reward pathways. The existence of bidirectional interactions between different drugs of abuse, such as opioids and cannabinoids, provides further findings to support this common neurobiological substrate for most drugs of abuse. Therefore, in spite of the different mechanisms of action, all the drugs of abuse produce neural dysregulations involving similar neurochemical and neuroanatomical pathways that are responsible for the initiation and maintenance of the drug addictive process.

References

Acquas E, Di Chiara G (1992) Depression of mesolimbic dopamine transmission and sensitization to morphine during opiate abstinence. J Neurochem 58: 1620–1625

Acquas E, Carboni E, Di Chiara G (1991) Profound depression of mesolimbic dopamine release after morphine withdrawal in dependent rats. Eur J Pharmacol 193: 133–134

Alheid GF, Heimer L (1988) New perspectives in basal forebrain organization of special relevance for neuropsychiatric disorders: the striatopallidal, amygdaloid, and corticopetal components of substantia innominata. Neuroscience 27: 1–39

Bourtchuladze R, Frenguelli B, Blendy J, Cioffi D, Schutz G, Silva AJ (1994) Deficient long-term memory in mice with a targeted mutation of the cAMP-responsive element-binding protein. Cell 79: 59–68

Braida D, Pozzi M, Parolaro D, Sala M (2001) Intracerebral self-administration of the cannabinoid receptor agonist CP 55:940 in the rat: interaction with the opioid system. Eur J Pharmacol 413: 227–234

Castañe A, Robledo P, Matifas A, Kieffer, Maldonado R (2003) Cannabinoid withdrawal syndrom is reduced in double mu and delta opioid receptor mice. Eur J Neurosci 17: 155–159

Chen J, Nye HE, Kelz MB, Hiroi N, Nakabeppu Y, Hope BT, Nestler EJ (1995) Regulation of delta FosB and FosB-like proteins by electroconvulsive seizure and cocaine treatments. Mol Pharmacol 48: 880–889

Chen JP, Paredes W, Lowinson JH, Gardner EL (1991) Strain-specific facilitation of dopamine efflux by delta-tetrahydrocannabinol in the nucleus accumbens of rat: an in vivo microdialysis study. Neurosci Lett 129: 136–180

Corrigall WA, Franklin KBJ, Coen KM, Clarke PBS (1992) The mesomlimbic dopaminergic system is implicated in the reinforcing effects of nicotine. Psycopharmacology 107: 285–289

Cummings S, Elde R, Ells J, Lindall A (1983) Corticotropin releasing factor immunoreactivity is widely distributed within the central nervous system of the rat: an immunohistochemical study. J Neurosci 3: 1355–1368

Di Chiara G, Imperato A (1988) Drug abused by humans preferentially increase synaptic dopamine concentrations in the mesolimbic system of freely moving rats. Proc Natl Acad Sci USA 94: 5274–5278

Diana M, Pistis M, Carboni S, Gessa GL, Rossetti ZL (1993) Profound decrement of mesolimbic dopaminergic neuronal activity during ethanol withdrawal syndrome in rats: electrophysiological and biochemical evidence. Proc Natl Acad Sci USA 90: 7966–7969

Diana M, Pistis M, Muntoni A, Gessa G (1996) Mesolimbic dopaminergic reduction outlasts ethanol withdrawal syndrome: evidence of protracted abstinence. Neuroscience 71: 411–415

Eckardt MJ, File SE, Gessa GL, Grant KA, Guerri C, Hoffman PL, Kalant H, Koob GF, Li TK, Tabakoff B (1998) Effects of moderate alcohol consumption on the central nervous system. Alcohol Clin Exp Res 22: 998–1040

Everitt BJ, Parkinson JA, Olmstead MC, Arroyo M, Robledo P, Robbins TW (1999) Associative processes in addiction and reward: the role of amygdala-ventral striatal subsystems. Ann NY Acad Sci 877: 412–438

Gessa GL, Melis M, Muntoni AL, Diana M (1998) Cannabinoids activate mesolimbic dopamine neurons by an action on cannabinoid CB1 receptors. Eur J Pharmacol 341: 39–44

Ghozland S, Matthes HW, Simonin F, Filliol D, Kieffer BL, Maldonado R (2002) Motivational effects of cannabinoids are mediated by mu-opioid and kappa-opioid receptors. J Neurosci 22: 1146–1154

Golberg SR, Munzar P, Justinova Z, Tanda G (2001) Effects of naltrexone on intravenous self-administration of delta-9-tetrahydrocannabinol (THC) by squirrel monkeys under fixed-ratio and second-order schedules. Int Cannab Res Soc Meeting, p 102

Grant S, London ED, Newlin DB, Villemagne VL, Liu X, Contoreggi C, Phillips RL, Kimes AS, Margolin A (1996) Activation of memory circuits during cue-elicited cocaine craving. Proc Natl Acad Sci USA 93: 12040–12045

Guitart X, Nestler EJ (1989) Identification of morphine- and cyclic AMP-regulated phosphoproteins (MARPPs) in the locus coeruleus and other regions of rat brain: regulation by acute and chronic morphine. J Neurosci 9: 4371–4387
Guitart X, Thompson MA, Mirante CK, Greenberg ME, Nestler EJ (1992) Regulation of cyclic AMP response element-binding protein (CREB) phosphorylation by acute and chronic morphine in the rat locus coeruleus. J Neurochem 58: 1168–1171
Heyser CJ, Roberts AJ, Schulteis G, Koob GF (1999) Central administration of an opiate antagonist decreses oral ethanol self-administration in rats. Alcohol Clin Exp Res 23: 1468–1476
Hilderbrand BE, Nomikos GG, Hertel P, Schilstrom B, Svensson TH (1998) Reduced dopamine output in the nucleus accumbens but not in the medial prefrontal cortex in rats displaying a mecamylamine-precipitated nicotine withdrawal syndrome. Brain Res 779: 214–225
Hine B, Friedman E, Torrelio M, Gershon S (1975a) Tetrahydrocanabinol-attenuated abstinence and induced rotation in morphine-dependent rats: possible involvement of dopamine. Neuropharmacology 14: 607–610
Hine B, Friedman E, Torrelio M, Gershon S (1975b) Morphine-dependent rats: blockade of precipitated abstinence by tetrahydrocannabinol. Science 187: 443–445
Hope BT, Nye HE, Kelz MB, Self DW, Iadarola MJ, Nakabeppu Y, Duman RS, Nestler EJ (1994) Induction of a long-lasting AP-1 complex composed of altered Fos-like proteins in brain by chronic cocaine and other chronic treatments. Neuron 13: 1235–1244
Howlett AC, Fleming RM (1984) Cannabinoid inhibition of adenyly cyclase. Pharmacoloby of the response in neuroblastoma cel membranes. Mol Pharmacol 27: 429–439
Hutcheson DM, Tzavara ET, Smadja C, Valjent E, Roques BP, Hanoune J, Maldonado R (1998) Behavioural and biochemical evidence for signs of abstinence in mice chronically treated with delta-9-tetrahydrocannabinol. Br J Pharmacol 125: 1567–1577
Hyman SE, Nestler EJ (1996) Initiation and adaptation: a paradigm for understanding psychotropic drug action. Am J Psychiatry 153: 151–162
Hyman SE, Malenka RC (2001) Addiction and the brain: the neurobiology of compulsion and its persistence. Nat Rev Neurosci 2: 695–703
Jaffe JH (1990) Trivializing dependence. Br J Addict 85: 1425–1427
Karin M, Liu Z, Zandi E (1997) AP-1 function and regulation. Curr Opin Cell Biol 9: 240–246
Kaymakcalan S, Ayhan IH, Tulunay FC (1977) Naloxone-induced or postwithdrawal abstinence signs in delta9-tetrahydrocannabinol-tolerant rats. Psychopharmacology 55: 243–249
Kelz MB, Nestler EJ (2000) deltaFosB: a molecular switch underlying long-term neural plasticity. Curr Opin Neurol 13: 715–720
Kelz MB, Chen J, Carlezon WA Jr, Whisler K, Gilden L, Beckmann AM, Steffen C, Zhang YJ, Marotti L, Self DW, Tkatch T, Baranauskas G, Surmeier DJ, Neve RL, Duman RS, Picciotto MR, Nestler EJ (1999) Expression of the transcription factor deltaFosB in the brain controls sensitivity to cocaine. Nature 401: 272–276
Koob G (1992) Drugs of abuse: anatomy, pharmacology and function of reward pathways. Trends Pharmacol Sci 13: 170–177
Koob GF (1996) Drug addiction: the yin and yang of hedonic homeostasis. Neuron 16: 893–896
Koob GF (1999) Cocaine reward and dopamine receptors: love at first site. Arch Gen Psychiatry 56: 1107–1108
Koob GF, Bloom FE (1988) Cellular and molecular mechanisms of drug dependence. Science 242: 715–723
Koob GF, Le Moal M (1997) Drug abuse: hedonic homeostatic dysregulation. Science 278: 52–58

Koob GF, LeMoal M (2001) Drug addiction, dysregulation of reward, and allostasis. Neuropsychopharmacology 24: 97–129
Koob GF, Stinus L, Le Moal M, Bloom FE (1989) Opponent process theory of motivation: neurobiological evidence from studies of opiate dependence. Neurosci Biobehav Rev 13: 135–140
Kreek MJ, Ragunath J, Plevy S, Hamer D, Schneider B, Hartman N (1984) ACTH, cortisol and beta-endorphin response to metyrapone testing during chronic methadone maintenance treatment in humans. Neuropeptides 5: 277–278
Ledent C, Valverde O, Cossu G, Petitet F, Aubert JF, Beslot F, Bohme GA, Imperato A, Pedrazzini T, Roques BP, Vassart G, Fratta W, Parmetier M (1999) Unresponsiveness to cannabinoids and reduced addictive effects of opiates in CB1 receptor knockout mice. Science 283: 15–19
Lichtman AH, Sheikh SM, Loh HH, Martin BR (2001) Opioid and cannabinoid modulation of precipitated withdrawal in delta(9)-tetrahydrocannabinol and morphine-dependent mice. J Pharmacol Exp Ther 298: 1007–1014
Lovinger DM, White G, Weight FF (1989) Ethanol inhibits NMDA-activated ion current in hippocampal neurons. Science 243: 1721–1724
Maldonado R (2003) Opioid system involvement in cannabinoid tolerance and dependence. In: Maldonado R (ed) Molecular biology of drug addiction. Humana Press, Totowa, pp 221–245
Maldonado R, Rodriguez de Fonseca F (2002) Cannabinoid addiction: behavioral models and neural correlates. J Neurosci 22: 3326–3331
Maldonado R, Stinus L, Gold LH, Koob GF (1992) Role of different brain structures in the expression of the physical morphine withdrawal syndrome. J Pharmacol Exp Ther 261: 669–677
Maldonado R, Blendy JA, Tzavara E, Gass P, Roques BP, Hanoune J, Schutz G (1996) Reduction of morphine abstinence in mice with a mutation in the gene encoding CREB. Science 273: 657–659
Martin M, Ledent C, Parmentier M, Maldonado R, Valverde O (2000) Cocaine but not morphine, induce conditioned place preference and sensitization to locomotor responses in CB-1 knockout mice. Eur J Neurosci 12: 4038–4046
Matthews RT, German DC (1984) Electrophysiological evidence for excitation of rat ventral tegmental area dopamine neurons by morphine. Neuroscience 11: 617–625
Mereu G, Fadda F, Gessa GL (1984) Ethanol stimulates the firing rate of nigral dopaminergic neurons in unanesthetized rats. Brain Res 292: 63–69
Mereu G, Kong-Woo PY, Boi V, Gessa GL, Naes L, Westfall TC (1987) Preferential stimulation of ventral tegmental dopaminergic neurons by nicotine. Eur J Pharmacol 141: 395–399
Merlo-Pick E, Lorang M, Yeganeh M, Rodriguez de Fonseca F, Raber J, Koob GF, Weiss F (1995) Increase of extracellular corticotropin-releasing factor-like immunoreactivity levels in the amygdala of awake rats during restraint stress and ethanol withdrawal as measured by microdialysis. J Neurosci 15: 5439–5447
Moratalla R, Elibol B, Vallejo M, Graybiel AM (1996) Network-level changes in expression of inducible Fos-Jun proteins in the striatum during chronic cocaine treatment and withdrawal. Neuron 17: 147–156
Navarro M, Chowen J, Rocio A, Carrera M, Del Arco I, Villanua MA, Martin Y, Roberts AJ, Koob GF, de Fonseca FR (1998) CB1 cannabinoid receptor antagonist-induced opiate withdrawal in morphine-dependent rats. Neuroreport 9: 3397–3402
Nestler EJ (2001) Molecular basis of long-term plasticity underlying addiction. Nat Rev Neurosci 2: 119–128
Nestler EJ, Tallman JF (1988) Chronic morphine treatment increases cyclic AMP-dependent protein kinase activity in the rat locus coeruleus. Mol Pharmacol 33: 127–132
Nestler EJ, Erdos JJ, Terwilliger R, Duman RS, Tallman JF (1989) Regulation of G proteins by chronic morphine in the rat locus coeruleus. Brain Res 476: 230–239

Nye HE, Nestler EJ (1996) Induction of chronic Fos-related antigens in rat brain by chronic morphine administration. Mol Pharmacol 49: 636–645
Nye HE, Hope BT, Kelz MB, Iadarola M, Nestler EJ (1995) Pharmacological studies of the regulation of chronic Fos-related antigen induction by cocaine in the striatum and nucleus accumbens. J Pharmacol Exp Ther 275: 1671–1680
Parsons LH, Smith AD, Justice JB Jr (1991) Basal extracellular dopamine is decreased in the rat nucleus accumbens during abstinence from chronic cocaine. Synapse 9: 60–65
Petit HO, Ettenberg A, Bloom FE, Koob GF (1984) Destruction of dopamine in the nucleus accumbens selectively attenuates cocaine but not heroin self-administration in rats. Psycopharmacology 84: 167–173
Pfeffer AO, Samson HH (1988) Haloperidol and apomorphine effects on ethanol reinforcement in free-feeding rats. Pharmacol Biochem Behav 29: 343–350
Picciotto M, Corrigal W (2002) Neuronal systems underlying behaviors related to nicotine addiction: neural circuits and molecular genetics. J Neurosci 22: 3338–3341
Pich EM, Pagliusi SR, Tessari M, Talabot-Ayer D, Hooft HR, Chiamulera C (1997) Common neural substrates for the addictive properties of nicotine and cocaine. Science 275: 83–86
Pontieri FE, Tanda G, Di Chiara G (1995) Intravenous cocaine, morphine, and amphetamine preferentially increase extra cellular dopamine in the "shell" as compared with the "core" of the rat nucleus accumbens. Proc Natl Acad Sci USA 92: 12304–12308
Pontieri FE, Tanda G, Di Chiara G (1996) Effects of nicotine on the nucleus accumbens and similarity to those of addictive drugs. Nature 382: 255–257
Richards G, Schoch P, Haefely W (1991) Benzodiazepine receptors: new vistas. Semin Neurosci 3: 191–203
Robbe D, Alonso G, Duchamp F, Bockaert J, Manzoni OJ (2001) Localization and mechanisms of action of cannabinoid receptors at the glutamatergic synapses of the mouse nucleus accumbens. J Neurosci 21: 109–116
Roberts AJ, McArthur RA, Hull EE, Post C, Koob GF (1998) Effects of amperozoide, 8-OH-DPAT, and FG 5974 on operant responding for ethanol. Psycopharmacology 137: 25–32
Roberts AJ, Heyser CJ, McDonald JS, Kieffer BL, Matthes HWD, Koob GF, Gold LH (2000) Mu opioid receptor knockout mice do not self-administer alcohol. J Pharmacol Exp Ther 293: 1002–1008
Robinson TE, Berridge KC (1993) The neural basis of drug craving: an incentive-sensitization theory of addiction. Brain Res Rev 18: 247–291
Rodriguez de Fonseca F, Carrera MRA, Navarro M, Koob GF, Weiss F (1997) Activation of corticotropin-releasing factor in the limbic system during cannabinoid withdrawal. Science 276: 2050–2054
Rossetti ZL, Hmaidan Y, Gessa GL (1992) Marked inhibition of mesolimbic dopamine release: a common feature of ethanol, morphine, cocaine and amphetamine abstinence in rats. Eur J Pharmacol 221: 227–234
Rubino T, Vigano D, Massi P, Parolaro D (2000a) Changes in the cannabinoid receptor binding, G protein coupling, and cyclic AMP cascade in the CNS of rats tolerant to and dependent on the synthetic cannabinoid compound CP55,940. J Neurochem 75: 2080–2086
Rubino T, Vigano' D, Massi P, Spinello M, Zagato E, Giagnoni G, Parolaro D (2000b) Chronic delta-9-tetrahydrocannabinol treatment increases cAMP levels and cAMP-dependent protein kinase activity in some rat brain regions. Neuropharmacology 39: 1331–1336
Rudnick G, Clark J (1993) From synapse to vesicle: the reuptake and storage of biogenic amine neurotransmitters. Biochim Biophys Acta 1144: 249–263
Ryabinin AE, Wang YM (1998) Repeated alcohol administration differentially affects c-Fos and FosB protein immunoreactivity in DBA/2J mice. Alcohol Clin Exp Res 22: 1646–1654

Schulteis G, Heyser CJ, Koob GF (1997) Opiate withdrawal signs precipitated by naloxone following a single exposure to morphine: potentiation with a second morphine treatment. Psychopharmacology 129: 56–65

Sharma SK, Klee WA, Nirenberg M (1975) Dual regulation of adenylate cyclase accounts for narcotic tolerance and dependence. Proc Natl Acad Sci USA 75: 3092–3096

Shippenberg TS, Herz A, Spanagel R, Bals-Kubik R, Stein C (1992) Conditioning of opioid reinforcement: neuroanatomical and neurochemical susbstrates. Ann NY Acad Sci 654: 347–356

Solomon RL, Corbit JD (1974) An apponent-process theory of motivation. I. Temporal dynamics of affect. Psychol Rev 81: 119–145

Tanda G, Pontieri FE, Di Chiara (1997) Cannabinoid and heroin activation of mesolimbic dopamine transmisi6n by a common mu1 opioid receptor mechanism. Science 276: 2048–2050

Tsou K, Brown S, Sañudo-Peña MC, Mackie K, Walker JM (1998) Immunohistochemical distribution of cannabinoid CB_1 receptors in the rat central nervous system. Neuroscience 83: 393–411

Tzavara ETH, Valjent E, Firmo C, Mas M, Beslot F, Defer N, Roques BP, Hanoune J, Maldonado R (2000) Cannabinoid withdrawal is dependent upon PKA activation in the cerebelum. Eur J Neurosci 12: 1038–1046

Ungless MA, Whistler JL, Malenka RC, Bonci A (2001) Single cocaine exposure in vivo induces long-term potentiation in dopamine neurons. Nature 411: 583–587

Valverde O, Maldonado R, Valjent E, Zimmer AM, Zimmer A (2000) Cannabinoid withdrawal syndrome is reduced in pre-proenkephalin knock-out mice. J Neurosci 20: 9284–9289

Valverde O, Noble F, Beslot F, Daugé V, Fournié-Zaluski MC, Roques BP (2001) Delta9-tetrahydrocannabinol releases and facilitates the effects of endogenous enkephalins: reduction in morphine withdrawal syndrome without change in rewarding effect. Eur J Neurosci 13: 1816–1824

Van Ree JM, Gerrits MA, Vanderschuren, LJ (1999) Opioids, reward and addiction: an encounter of biology, psychology, and medicine. Pharmacol Rev 51: 341–396

Vela G, Ruiz-Gayo M, Fuentes JA (1995) Anandamide decreases naloxone-precipitated withdrawal signs in mice chronically treated with morphine. Neuropharmacology 34: 665–668

Volkow ND, Fowler JS (2000) Addiction, a disease of compulsion and drive: involvement of the orbitofrontal cortex. Cerebral Cortex 10: 318–325

White FJ (1996) Synaptic regulation of mesocorticolimbic dopamine neurons. Annu Rev Neurosci 19: 405–436

Wise RA (1996) Addictive drugs and brains timulation reward. Annu Rev Neurosci 19: 319–340

Zimmer A, Valjent E, Konig M, Zimmer AM, Robledo P, Hahn H, Valverde O, Maldonado R (2001) Absence of delta-9-tetrahydrocannabinol dysphoric effects in dynorphin-deficient mice. J Neurosci 21: 9499–9505

Author's address: Dr. R. Maldonado, Laboratori de Neurofarmacologia, Facultat de Cienc̀es de la Salut i de la Vida, Universitat Pompeu Fabra, C/Dr Aiguador 80, E-08003 Barcelona, Spain, e-mail: rafael.maldonado@cexs.upf.es

Biological markers in alcoholism

A. Helander

Department of Clinical Neuroscience, Karolinska Institutet & Hospital, Stockholm, Sweden

Summary. Alcohol biomarkers include tests indicative of acute or chronic alcohol consumption (state markers), and markers of a genetic predisposition to develop alcohol dependence after chronic exposure (trait markers). While a comprehensive trait marker for alcohol dependence has not been identified, a number of successful state markers for monitoring drinking status are used clinically. These tests provide direct or indirect ways to estimate the amounts of alcohol consumed and the duration of ingestion, and to detect any harmful effects on body functions resulting from long-term misuse. The most obvious method to prove recent drinking is by demonstrating the presence of ethanol in body fluids or breath, but, because ethanol is cleared fairly rapidly from the body, this method is limited to detect only very recent drinking. Measurement of urinary 5-hydroxytryptophol or ethyl glucuronide provide more sensitive methods to disclose recent drinking, because their washout constants are much longer than for ethanol. The liver functions test (GGT, AST and ALT in serum) and the mean corpuscular volume of erythrocytes (MCV) are among the standard diagnostic tools used to identify chronic alcohol exposure. The main disadvantage with these measures is that they have low sensitivity for recent excessive intake, and that raised levels may result from several causes besides heavy drinking, implying a low specificity for alcohol. Carbohydrate-deficient transferrin (CDT), which refers to changes in the carbohydrate composition of serum transferrin, is a more specific marker for identifying excessive alcohol consumption and monitoring abstinence during outpatient treatment. The alcohol biomarkers improves knowledge of drinking patterns in both individuals and populations, and they are also valuable tools for the objective evaluation of treatment efforts. Alcohol markers have, for example, found uses in early identification of at-risk and harmful drinking, and they help to monitor abstinence and relapse in response to outpatient treatment.

Introduction

Biological markers in alcoholism include markers indicative of recent (acute or chronic) alcohol consumption or subsequent alcohol-induced organ damage ("state markers") but also markers of a genetic predisposition to develop dependence on alcohol after chronic exposure ("trait markers"). It is well-known that addictive disorders tend to run in families. Twin and adoption studies, as well as more recent molecular genetic research, have consistently confirmed that the risk for onset of alcohol dependence is genetically influenced, explaining approximately half of the risk. An intensive search for trait markers has generated a large number of candidate neurochemical, electrophysiological and personality characteristics, and genes showing association with alcohol dependence. Promising results have, for example, been obtained in studies on the platelet serotonin transporter, activities of monoamine oxidase (MAO) B and adenylyl cyclase enzymes, dopamine receptor polymorphisms (e.g., DRD2), and EEG alpha-wave activity (Enoch and Goldman, 2001; Ratsma et al., 2002; Schuckit, 2000). However, published data have sometimes been conflicting (DRD2) (Gelernter et al., 1993) and some candidates were later suggested not to be state independent; i.e., their reliability as trait markers may be diminished by factors such as recent alcohol consumption (adenylyl cyclase) (Hoffman et al., 2002) or smoking (MAO-B) (Coccini et al., 2002). Another problem is that like many other common, complex disease states, alcohol dependence is assumed to be multifactorial in that polygenetic and environmental factors combine together. So far, the only clear-cut genetic association with risk for alcohol use and abuse is in the functional polymorphisms of the alcohol dehydrogenase (ADH) and aldehyde dehydrogenase (ALDH) enzymes. Individuals with an inactive form of mitochondrial ALDH (ALDH2*2), which is found in Oriental populations, possess an inborn "disulfiram-like" aversive effect to alcohol and are thereby discouraged from excessive drinking and hence protected from developing dependence (Agarwal, 1997). On the other hand, individuals with the heterozygous ALDH2*1/2*2 genotype who do drink alcohol are at higher risk for developing alcohol-related liver damage and cancers than those with the homozygous, active ALDH2*1/2*1 genotype (Higuchi et al., 1995; Yokoyama et al., 2001).

While a comprehensive trait marker for a familial genetic predisposition to develop alcohol dependence has yet to be identified, a number of successful state markers for the detection and monitoring of drinking status are used clinically (Fig. 1). This paper gives a survey of conventional and candidate state markers of alcohol use and abuse and also highlights some clinical applications.

Identification of alcohol use and abuse

Activities attempted at early identification and intervention of individuals with harmful levels of alcohol consumption can be justified for several reasons. Alcohol-related problems are common in the Western world, and they are typically associated with negative medical, social, and economical consequences to both the individual and society. Excess drinking is a common contributing risk factor in sickness, accidents, injury and trauma, and a leading

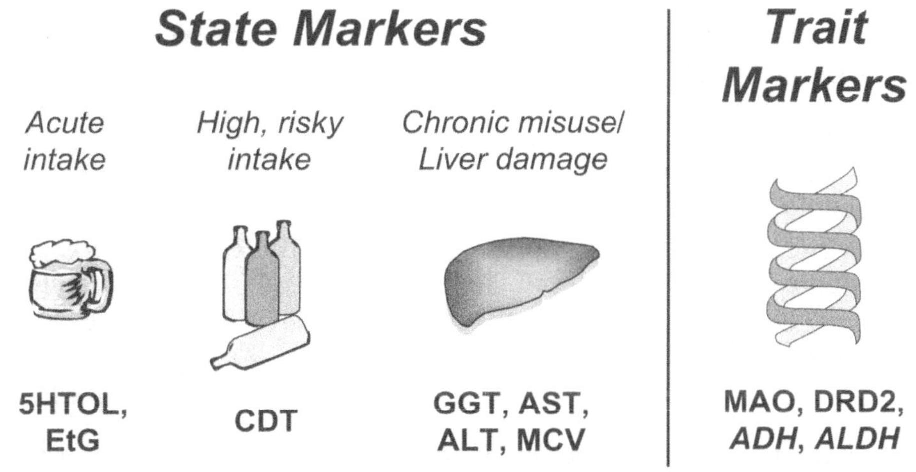

Fig. 1. Alcohol biomarkers include tests indicative of acute or chronic consumption or alcohol-induced organ damage (state markers), and candidate markers of a genetic predisposition to develop alcohol dependence after chronic exposure (trait markers). While a comprehensive trait marker for alcohol dependence has not been identified, a number of successful state markers for monitoring drinking status are used clinically

cause of premature deaths (Cherpitel, 1997). Alcohol is also an important predictor of criminal activity, personal violence, and property damage (Shepherd, 1994). Hence, several studies have recommended use of random screening for alcohol-related problems, and testing on suspicion, in primary care, hospital, and workplace settings, to enable treatment to be initiated prior to the development of actual symptoms (D'Onofrio and Degutis, 2002; Hermansson et al., 2000; Reid et al., 1999).

The traditional and most objective way ("gold standard") to test for intake of alcohol is to determine the presence of ethanol in body fluids or breath (Jones, 1995). However, this method is limited to detect only very recent drinking, because ethanol is cleared fairly rapidly from the body with resulting poor sensitivity. Accordingly, a person may consume considerable amounts of alcohol in the evening and still present a negative ethanol test result the following morning (Bendtsen et al., 1998). Furthermore, finding a single sample positive for ethanol is not usually a reliable indication of the person's drinking habits or whether there might be underlying problems.

Verbal measures such as clinical interviews and screening instruments (e.g., the AUDIT, CAGE, and MAST) are often employed to obtain data about a person's alcohol consumption (Reid et al., 1999). Although detailed quantity–frequency interviews (e.g., Timeline Followback) represent an important source of information and typically have a low rate of false-positive responses, the primary weakness is that people may not report their alcohol intake accurately (Midanik, 1988). There are also indications that persons who are dependent on alcohol underreport their true intake more than light-to-moderate drinkers (Fuller et al., 1988; Helander et al., 1999). Therefore, as the clinical signs of heavy drinking are rather unreliable, at least in the early stages of misuse, under-diagnosis of alcohol abuse and dependence is not uncommon when relying solely on self-reports of alcohol use.

To assist physicians with detecting at-risk and harmful drinking in a more objective way, a wide variety of biological state markers based on measurements of direct and indirect effects of alcohol consumption on blood and urine chemistry and haematology have been proposed, and there is a continuous development of new candidates for clinical evaluation. The alcohol biomarkers furnish ways to estimate roughly the amounts consumed and the duration of ingestion (e.g., acute or chronic heavy drinking), and evaluate any harmful effects on the body as a result of prolonged misuse (e.g., alcohol-induced liver injury).

Sensitivity, specificity, and predictive values of biological markers

Biological markers are evaluated in terms of diagnostic sensitivity and specificity. In this context, sensitivity refers to the ability of the test to detect those individuals with a certain level and/or duration of alcohol consumption, whereas specificity refers to the ability to exclude those who drink less. Consequently, a highly sensitive marker yields few false-negative results and one with high specificity few false positives. The ideal marker should be both 100% sensitive and 100% specific but this is hardly ever achieved. Instead, because of biological heterogeneity within and between individuals both at baseline and in response to a given alcohol dose, there is usually an overlap between reference intervals for "normal" and "abnormal" values, yielding a diagnostic grey zone. Some people may be able to drink excessively without displaying abnormal test results, which implies a low sensitivity of the marker in these subjects. On the other hand, some alcohol markers may yield abnormal values also in people suffering from non-alcohol related problems, or after taking certain kinds of medication, which implies a low specificity.

Reference intervals for laboratory parameters are commonly calculated as the mean ± 2 times the standard deviation (SD) of values in a well-defined healthy control population. Assuming a Gaussian distribution, this practice will always result in a specificity of less than 100% because 5% of the control values will be lying outside the upper and lower reference limits. There are certain factors that need to be considered when establishing reference intervals for alcohol biomarkers. First, a limitation is that many studies evaluating the sensitivity and specificity of biological alcohol markers have relied solely on self-report data as the gold standard about alcohol consumption. Considering that many patients fail to provide an accurate history of their true intake, this creates a validity problem. Second, alcohol consumption patterns and social drinking norms vary between cultures and societies, and thereby also the constitution of "healthy control" populations. The use of receiver-operating characteristic (ROC) curves, where the relation between sensitivity and specificity at different cut-offs between normal and abnormal values are evaluated, has become a popular tool for comparing the diagnostic performances of alcohol markers and selecting optimal threshold limits (Zweig and

Campbell, 1993). However, such studies should preferably focus on the sensitivity at the higher specificity range, and not on the total area-under-the-ROC curve because this covers the entire specificity range from 0 to 100%, most of which is of very limited use in clinical practice.

In routine use, the likelihood of obtaining a correct classification ("predictive values") with a biological alcohol marker is strongly related to the prevalence of alcohol use/abuse in the population to be studied. The positive predictive value (PPV) gives the proportion of truly positive test results out of all positive results (i.e., out of the sum of true and false positives), and the negative predictive value (NPV) the proportion of truly negative test result out of all negative results (sum of true and false negatives). Also when using a marker with fairly high sensitivity and specificity, the risk for incorrect classification might be rather high if the impairment occurs only infrequently in the study population. Accordingly, markers used to detect excessive alcohol consumption will perform better (higher PPV) in studies on selected, high-risk populations (e.g., drunk drivers) than on the general population.

The sensitivity, specificity, and predictive values of biological markers are highly influenced by the cut-off, or decision, limit chosen do distinguish between a normal and an abnormal value. For example, the reference interval may be adjusted to obtain a higher specificity of the test, but at the same time the sensitivity becomes reduced, and vice versa. If an alcohol marker is to be used for general screening of potentially harmful drinking levels or early detection of relapse in connection with rehabilitation as outpatients, this places especially high demands on the sensitivity. Many screening tests used in primary care have a low PPV. Cancer markers, for example, show a high false-positive rate, because the preliminary screening step must be very sensitive to include as many as possible of those with the disease for subsequent re-testing with a more specific confirmatory assay (e.g., biopsy). In contrast, if a positive result for an alcohol biomarker may lead to legal sanctions to the individual, such as loss of employment or revocation of driving license, this places high demands on the specificity, as reflected in a low risk for obtaining false-positive identifications.

Laboratory tests of acute alcohol consumption

Ethanol

The most obvious method to prove recent intake of alcohol is by demonstrating the presence of ethanol in body fluids (blood, urine, or saliva) or breath (Jones, 1995). Determination of ethanol is a relatively simple task and reliable results can be obtained with gas-chromatographic or enzymatic methods (Jones and Schuberth, 1989). For some field applications (e.g., in traffic medicine, hospital emergency room settings, and workplace testing), non-invasive sampling methods may be feasible to monitor alcohol exposure such as analysing expired air with hand-held breathalysers or saliva with dip-sticks (Bendtsen et al., 1999; Smolle et al., 1999). Compared with blood and breath, ethanol can usually be detected for some hours longer in urine, owing to retention of urine in the bladder (Helander et al., 1996a).

The ingested ethanol is rapidly absorbed from the stomach and small intestine into the circulatory system and distributes in all body fluids and tissues in proportion to the water content. Ethanol is cleared fairly rapidly at a rate of about 0.1 g/kg per hour (corresponding to 0.15–0.20 g/L per hour in the blood), primarily due to metabolism in the liver, with even more rapid elimination noted in heavy drinkers. As a consequence, a person may consume substantial amounts of alcohol in the evening (at least one bottle of wine, or ~4–5 cans of beer, or ~5–6 drinks, corresponding to ~60–80 g ethanol) and still present a negative ethanol test the following morning (Bendtsen et al., 1998). Indeed, there are indications that individuals undergoing outpatient treatment for drug-related problems often drink alcohol without admitting to, but they regulate the amount consumed and also the time they stop drinking in the evening to be able to present a negative ethanol result at the time for testing (Helander et al., 1999).

A positive ethanol test may and may not have any relationship to chronic misuse, because a low concentration of ethanol could result from very recent intake of a small alcohol dose as well as from the late stages of eliminating a much larger intoxicating dose. However, finding a high ethanol concentration during daytime clearly indicates advanced drinking habits, and showing little or no signs of intoxication even at a fairly high ethanol concentration indicates that the person has become tolerant to ethanol as a result of prolonged excessive exposure. Checking for a positive ethanol concentration is therefore always advisable.

Ethyl glucuronide (EtG)

Besides the two-stage oxidation process of ethanol via ADH and ALDH mainly in the liver that accounts for at least 95% of total ethanol elimination, a very small fraction (<0.1%) (Dahl et al., 2002) of the ingested dose undergoes conjugation with UDP-glucuronic acid to produce ethyl glucuronide (EtG), a water soluble metabolite which is excreted in the urine (Jaakonmaki et al., 1967; Schmitt et al., 1997). During recent years, the development of improved analytical methods based on mass spectrometry (GC–MS and LC–MS) has renewed the interest in this ethanol metabolite as a biological alcohol marker (Nishikawa et al., 1999; Schmitt et al., 1995; Stephanson et al., 2002).

EtG is of interest as a marker of acute alcohol consumption mainly because the washout constant is much longer than for ethanol with resulting higher sensitivity (Dahl et al., 2002; Schmitt et al., 1997). Being a direct metabolite of ethanol, EtG is also indicated to be very specific for alcohol intake (Seidl et al., 2001). Determination of EtG in blood and urine thus provides a means to determine if a person has recently consumed alcohol, even for many hours after the ingested ethanol dose has already been eliminated. However, recent studies have demonstrated that the concentration of EtG in urine can be lowered markedly by drinking large amounts of water prior to voiding, whereas this strategy does not influence the EtG/creatinine ratio, nor the concentration of ethanol (Dahl et al., 2002). Accordingly, in line with the routines for urine testing of drugs-of-abuse (George and Braithwaite, 1995), expressing urinary EtG as a ratio to creatinine may be recommended to compensate for urine dilution, although even this strategy will not be useful once the EtG concentration has become diluted to below the limit of detection of the analytical method. Intentional dilution of the urine by drinking large volumes of fluid prior to sampling will thus remain a way to shorten the detection time of this new alcohol marker.

Ratio of 5-hydroxytryptophol to 5-hydroxyindole-3-acetic acid (5HTOL/5HIAA)

Ethanol ingestion is known to interfere with the metabolism of serotonin (5-hydroxytryptamine) and this interaction can be utilized for indirect detection of recent alcohol consumption. 5-Hydroxytryptophol (5HTOL) is normally a minor serotonin metabolite in the urine (<1%) but during ethanol metabolism the formation of 5HTOL increases dramatically in a dose-dependent manner, whereas 5-hydroxyindole-3-acetic acid (5HIAA), the major metabolite under normal conditions (>99%), is correspondingly decreased (Davis et al., 1967; Helander et al., 1993). This shift in serotonin metabolism occurs because of competitive inhibition of ALDH by acetaldehyde, the intermediate metabolite of ethanol oxidation via ADH, and the change in redox state to a more reduced potential during ethanol metabolism (Svensson et al., 1999). The urinary output of 5HTOL does not recover to baseline levels until several hours after ethanol is no longer measurable (Helander et al., 1993). Accordingly, as also observed for EtG, measuring 5HTOL in urine provides a much more sensitive method for disclosing recent drinking than testing for ethanol and can detect intake of even moderate amounts of alcohol within the past ~24 hours (Helander et al., 1996a, 1999).

To improve the accuracy of this acute alcohol marker in clinical use, 5HTOL should be expressed as a ratio to urinary 5HIAA instead of creatinine. This practice will compensate for variations in the 5HTOL concentration caused by urine dilution, dietary intake of serotonin (high amounts in banana) (Helander et al., 1992), as well as treatment with antidepressant drugs (SSRI and MAOI) (Helander and Eriksson, 2002). Apart from alcohol consumption, disulfiram (Antabuse) therapy, which is a potent inhibitor of ALDH, represents the only known cause of a raised 5HTOL/5HIAA ratio (Beck et al., 1995). The baseline value for the urinary 5HTOL/5HIAA ratio is not influenced by prolonged excessive alcohol exposure and this marker can therefore be used to identify recent intake of alcohol in both social and chronic consumers.

5HTOL is excreted in the urine mainly in conjugated form with glucuronic acid (Helander et al., 1995). Determination of free 5HTOL can be performed by GC–MS after enzymatic hydrolysis (Voltaire et al., 1992) but 5HTOL may also be determined in the conjugated form (GTOL) by LC–MS. A direct immunoassay for GTOL is underway which will improve the utility of this marker in routine use. 5HIAA can be determined by HPLC with electrochemical detection (Helander et al., 1991).

Laboratory tests of chronic alcohol exposure

Conventional alcohol markers (GGT, AST, ALT, and MCV)

The conventional biochemical markers used to identify chronic alcohol exposure include the liver functions test gamma-glutamyltransferase (GGT) and aspartate and alanine aminotransferase (AST and ALT) in serum, and the mean corpuscular volume of erythrocytes (MCV) (Chick et al., 1981). GGT, AST and ALT are standard diagnostic tools used in clinical medicine (blood-chemistry panels) to indicate non-specific liver dysfunction, and MCV is often measured as part of a routine blood count.

A limitation with these measures is that they will mainly identify those persons who have already been drinking excessively for a considerable period of time (months–years), implying a low sensitivity for recent excessive alcohol intake. Another disadvantage is that they exhibit low specificity for alcohol, as raised levels may also result from several causes besides heavy drinking, including commonly prescribed drugs such as barbiturates and antiepileptics, factors such as smoking, obesity, and pregnancy, and most liver disorders of non-alcoholic origin (Aubin et al., 1998; Nilssen and Førde, 1994; Rosalki and Rau, 1972). Notably, coffee intake has been reported to inhibit the induction of liver enzymes caused by alcohol consumption, and may thus possibly protect against liver damage resulting from heavy drinking (Tanaka et al., 1998).

Due to their low sensitivity and specificity, the utility of the conventional alcohol markers may be limited in screening for hazardous or harmful drinking in the general population, but they are often helpful for follow-up of patients with already diagnosed alcohol-related liver affection. Furthermore, to date most causes of false-positive test results are well-known and can often be corrected for in the clinical situation.

Carbohydrate-deficient transferrin (CDT)

The iron-transport glycoprotein transferrin has two binding sites for iron and two oligosaccharide chains of complex structure. "Carbohydrate-deficient transferrin" (CDT), which refers to changes in the carbohydrate composition of these chains and, hence, in the isoform profile of serum transferrin, has proven useful as a biochemical marker for identifying excessive alcohol consumption and monitoring abstinence during outpatient treatment (Allen et al., 1994; Stibler, 1991). The most abundant transferrin isoform contains two biantennary carbohydrate chains with a total of four terminal sialic acid residues (named tetrasialotransferrin). However, individuals who have been

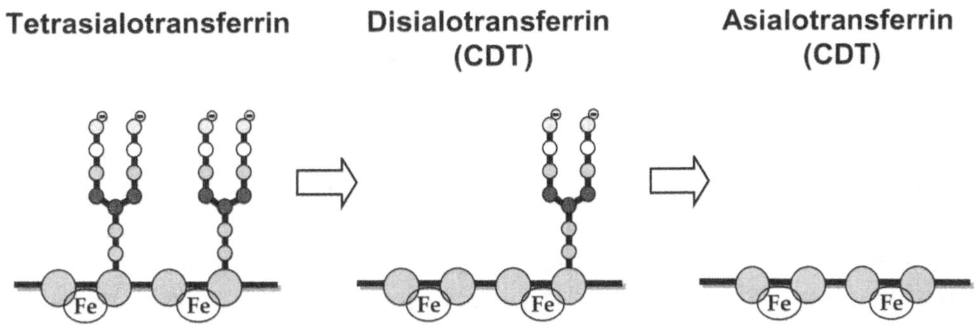

Fig. 2. Carbohydrate-deficient transferrin (CDT) is a specific biochemical marker for recent excessive alcohol consumption. The most abundant isoform of serum transferrin contains two biantennary carbohydrate chains with a total of four terminal, negatively charged sialic acid residues (tetrasialotransferrin). Individuals who have been drinking excessively over the past 2 or more weeks often show an increased level of CDT, corresponding to transferrin molecules that lack one (disialotransferrin) or both (asialotransferrin) of the carbohydrate chains

drinking at least 50–80g ethanol per day on average over the past 2 or more weeks often show an increased level of transferrin molecules that lack one (disialotransferrin) or both (asialotransferrin) of the carbohydrate chains (Fig. 2) (Landberg et al., 1995; Peter et al., 1998). The absence of negatively charged sialic acids results in a higher isoelectric point than for the major isoform tetrasialotransferrin, and most analytical procedures therefore utilize charge-based separation of the CDT molecules prior to quantification. When drinking is discontinued, the serum CDT level normalizes with a half-life of ~2 weeks (Jeppsson et al., 1993) and the time for return to within the reference interval could require one month or longer (Helander and Carlsson, 1996). The exact cause of the alcohol-induced elevation of CDT has still not been identified in detail.

Compared with the conventional laboratory methods used in routine clinical medicine to indicate prolonged excessive drinking, such as measures of liver damage, several studies have indicated that CDT enable detection to be made substantially earlier. However, it appears that the major value of CDT over the conventional tests is not a much higher sensitivity (Conigrave et al., 2002) but, rather, that it can, with better precision, differentiate between alcohol and other causes, such as non-alcohol liver disease (Meerkerk et al., 1998). Reported causes for false positive and false negative CDT results in the identification of alcohol abuse are mostly rare and include genetic transferrin D and B variants and advanced non-alcoholic liver disease (DiMartini et al., 2001; Helander et al., 2001). Increases in serum CDT are also observed in congenital disorders of glycosylation (CDG) (Helander et al., 2001; Stibler, 1991), an extremely rare, inherited neurological disorder which is often associated with variable mental retardation (Freeze, 2001). It should be recognized that the risk for incorrect determination of CDT is dependent in part on the choice of analytical method (Helander et al., 2001).

Several different procedures are currently applied for the routine measurement of serum CDT, but the transferrin isoforms covered and, hence, the definition of CDT, vary between tests (Arndt, 2001; Helander et al., 2001). The immunological assays are convenient and time-efficient for routine use in central laboratories with a high specimen throughput. However, a drawback with the current immunoassays is that they require an initial, time-consuming separation step of the CDT isoforms on minicolumns prior to quantification (Helander, 1999). The major advantage of methods based on HPLC and capillary electrophoresis, albeit being more laborious, is their ability to identify the genetic transferrin variants that may cause incorrect determination of CDT with the immunoassays. Ongoing activities aiming for an international standardisation of definitions, and harmonisation of procedures, for CDT, including the development of a reference method based on HPLC technique, are important factors to support advances in the use of CDT as a sensitive and specific alcohol marker (Helander et al., 2001).

Clinical application of biological alcohol markers

Use of alcohol biomarkers in primary care settings

In primary care settings, there is a need for simple and reliable methods to identify patients with alcohol-related problems in the first place (McQuade et al., 2000). Hitherto, testing for harmful and hazardous drinking has mainly employed the conventional laboratory parameters of liver damage included in routine blood-chemistry panels. Because these tests are not very specific for alcohol resulting in a high risk for false positive identifications, their usefulness for screening in the general population is limited. Another drawback is that they will mainly identify those who have already been drinking excessively for long periods, because alcohol-related liver affection is an end-stage of this process. The CDT test has also been evaluated for the same purpose, but, despite being more specific for alcohol, its accuracy for early identification of alcohol misuse in general practice has been questioned (Aertgeerts et al., 2001; Meerkerk et al., 1999). However, it is assumed that the ongoing standardisation and harmonisation of CDT procedures, including the development of a sensitive reference method, and use of more reliable, up-to-date CDT assays, will improve the utility of this marker in studies on unselected populations (Helander et al., 2001).

A number of workplace studies have provided evidence that screening for at-risk and harmful drinking with the use of instruments like CDT and the AUDIT questionnaire, combined with brief intervention, delivered as part of routine company health care may reduce alcohol consumption (Hermansson et al., 2000; Reid et al., 1999). To be well accepted by the employees, alcohol screening may be incorporated into the context of longitudinal health care programs, such as for high cholesterol and hypertension, in connection with routine health check-ups (Hermansson et al., 1998). Thereby, the screening will focus mainly on risk reduction (i.e., personal health) instead of detection of abuse or dependence.

Use of alcohol biomarkers in hospital settings

Many persons admitted to general hospitals have undiagnosed alcohol problems and may partly be treated for the consequences of their drinking (Carrigan et al., 2000; Hearne et al., 2002). Based on a positive ethanol test on admission, the prevalence of alcohol involvement among trauma patients has been found be 15–25% (Cherpitel et al., 1999) and even higher (>30%) during evening and late-night hours (Holt et al., 1980). Excessive drinkers often develop alcohol withdrawal syndrome and are therefore at increased risk for post-operative morbidity (e.g., sepsis, pneumonia, and bleeding) and mortality (Eggers et al., 2002; Martin et al., 2002). Identification and detoxification of patients with underlying alcohol-related problems prior to surgery can thus reduce the incidence of post-operative complications with need for extended, costly hospitalisation (Spies et al., 1996; Tønnesen, 1999). Recent studies have found the CDT test to be useful for this purpose (Spies et al., 1998; Tønnesen et al., 1999). Additionally, alcohol-dependent patients often continue to consume alcohol until just prior to surgery, and combining CDT with a sensitive short-term marker, such as the 5HTOL/5HIAA ratio in urine, could improve further the possibility to identify these high-risk patients at an early stage (Spies et al., 1999).

Use of alcohol biomarkers in rehabilitation of alcohol-dependent subjects

Biochemical alcohol markers are useful in monitoring adherence to treatment and early detection of relapse during outpatient treatment of alcohol-dependent subjects (Helander et al., 1996b; Huseby et al., 1997; Voltaire Carlsson et al., 1993). Because the response of different markers to excessive drinking may diverge considerably between individuals, the most sensitive single test can be identified by following changes in a set of complementary markers during a period of alcohol withdrawal (e.g., hospitalisation or disulfiram treatment) (Helander and Carlsson, 1996). In certain patients, GGT actually shows higher sensitivity for recent excessive drinking than CDT and the combined use of these two markers has therefore been recommended (Helander et al., 1996b). After discharge from inpatient treatment, serial testing could be continued on a routine or random basis, for example in connection with return visits to the clinic. A test to monitor acute alcohol consumption may also be employed in parallel. The urinary 5HTOL/5HIAA ratio, being much more sensitive than conventional breath or blood ethanol testing, has proven valuable for this purpose during outpatient treatment and can detect the occasional lapses that typically precedes a relapse (Fig. 3) (Helander et al., 1999).

During serial sampling, a rising test value may indicate return to drinking even before the relapse is detected by the physician's clinical diagnosis or

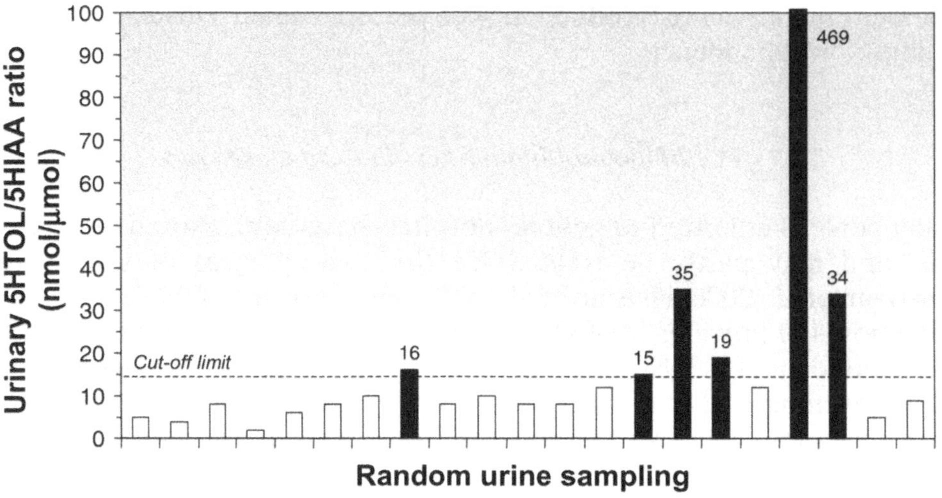

Fig. 3. Measurement of the urinary 5-hydroxytryptophol to 5-hydroxyindole-3-acetic acid ratio (5HTOL/5HIAA) provides a sensitive method to disclose recent drinking within the past ~24 hours, even for several hours after the ethanol is no longer measurable. During outpatient treatment, testing for acute alcohol consumption has proven valuable to detect occasional lapses that typically precede a relapse (the 5HTOL/5HIAA cut-off limit to indicate any recent drinking is <15 nmol/μmol)

admitted by the patient (Mitchell et al., 1997; Rosman et al., 1995). This practice can be improved further by introducing individualized instead of population-based reference limits between normal and elevated values (Borg et al., 1995; Irwin et al., 1988). This strategy will also increase the reliability of test results (a higher specificity), as some people have baseline values outside the reference interval even without prior excessive drinking. Giving patients feedback about the test results, for example in a graph, may improve self-report of alcohol intake and long-term treatment outcome (Helander et al., 1996b; Kristenson et al., 2002).

Legal applications for alcohol biomarkers

There are several legal applications for markers of alcohol use and abuse. In traffic medicine, they may aid in the identification of alcohol-dependent subjects among those being convicted for drunk driving (Iffland, 1996; Staak and Iffland, 1992). CDT in combination with GGT has also proven effective in confirmation of abstinence and detection of relapse in connection with rehabilitation of drunk drivers and regranting of driving licenses, and their use may reduce recidivism rates after relicensing (Kristenson and Jeppsson, 1998).

In forensic toxicology, testing for the 5HTOL/5HIAA ratio or EtG can be used to settle whether the ethanol identified in a blood or urine specimen originates from alcohol ingestion prior to death or has been generated artifactually (i.e., post mortem) (Helander et al., 1995). It is well-known that ethanol may be formed in the body between time of death and autopsy due to microbial action, and upon incorrect storage of unpreserved biological specimens prior to analysis (Jones et al., 1999). Accordingly, these markers of acute alcohol intake have also found uses in connection with the prosecution of drunk drivers, because challenging the results of forensic ethanol analysis due to contamination or artifactual formation is common (Jones and Helander, 1998).

Testing for acute alcohol consumption may also be applied in certain workplaces upon return to safety-sensitive duties (Hagan and Helander, 1997), because it is known that the acute and post-intoxication effects (hangover, fatigue) of heavy drinking will impair performance, resulting in an increased risk for accidents and injury (Dorafshar et al., 2002; Ragland et al., 2002; Wiese et al., 2000; Yesavage et al., 1994).

Conclusions

State markers of alcohol use and abuse provide direct and indirect ways to estimate roughly the amounts of alcohol consumed and the duration of ingestion, and to detect any harmful effects on body functions resulting from long-term misuse. The field of biochemical alcohol markers has expanded greatly over the years and both clinical and forensic applications are now well documented. When used properly, alcohol biomarkers improves knowledge of drinking patterns in both individuals and populations, and they are valuable tools for the objective evaluation of treatment efforts. However, there are a number of clinical and technical issues that need to be considered (Table 1),

Table 1. Clinical and analytical issues to be considered when choosing the appropriate alcohol marker for different purposes

Issue	Comments
Acute and/or chronic drinking?	— Does testing aim to detect recent acute or chronic drinking and/or any harmful effects of long-term misuse? — Should testing involve a single marker or a combination of complementary tests?
Time delay between drinking and sampling?	— What is the biological half-life of the marker? — How often should testing be repeated during follow-up?
Sensitivity, specificity, and predictive values?	— What is the likelihood of obtaining a correct identification in the population to be studied? — What cut-off limit should be applied — should focus be on high sensitivity or high specificity? — Does a positive test result need to be verified by a more specific confirmatory assay?
Ease of use and availability?	— Is the biological sample used for measurement easily accessible? — Is testing performed at the clinical central laboratory, or does it require a special laboratory? — What is the time to obtain the test result? — What is the cost of testing?

to improve the accuracy of alcohol markers for screening in unselected populations and follow-up of alcohol-dependent individuals during outpatient treatment.

References

Aertgeerts B, Buntinx F, Ansoms S, Fevery J (2001) Screening properties of questionnaires and laboratory tests for the detection of alcohol abuse or dependence in a general practice population. Br J Gen Pract 51: 206–217

Agarwal DP (1997) Molecular genetic aspects of alcohol metabolism and alcoholism. Pharmacopsychiatry 30: 79–84

Allen JP, Litten RZ, Anton RF, Cross GM (1994) Carbohydrate-deficient transferrin as a measure of immoderate drinking: remaining issues. Alcohol Clin Exp Res 18: 799–812

Arndt T (2001) Carbohydrate-deficient transferrin as a marker of chronic alcohol abuse: a critical review of preanalysis, analysis, and interpretation. Clin Chem 47: 13–27

Aubin HJ, Laureaux C, Zerah F, Tilikete S, Vernier F, Vallat B, Barrucand D (1998) Joint influence of alcohol, tobacco, and coffee on biological markers of heavy drinking in alcoholics. Biol Psychiatry 44: 638–643

Beck O, Helander A, Carlsson S, Borg S (1995) Changes in serotonin metabolism during treatment with the aldehyde dehydrogenase inhibitors disulfiram and cyanamide. Pharmacol Toxicol 77: 323–326

Bendtsen P, Jones AW, Helander A (1998) Urinary excretion of methanol and 5-hydroxytryptophol as biochemical markers of recent drinking in the hangover state. Alcohol Alcohol 33: 431–438

Bendtsen P, Hultberg J, Carlsson M, Jones AW (1999) Monitoring ethanol exposure in a clinical setting by analysis of blood, breath, saliva, and urine. Alcohol Clin Exp Res 23: 1446–1451

Borg S, Helander A, Voltaire Carlsson A, Högström-Brandt A-M (1995) Detection of relapses in alcohol dependent patients using carbohydrate-deficient transferrin: improvement with individualized reference levels during long-term monitoring. Alcohol Clin Exp Res 19: 961–963

Carrigan TD, Field H, Illingworth RN, Gaffney P, Hamer DW (2000) Toxicological screening in trauma. J Accid Emerg Med 17: 33–37

Cherpitel CJ (1997) Alcohol and violence-related injuries in the emergency room. Rec Dev Alcohol 13: 105–118

Cherpitel CJ, Giesbrecht N, Macdonald S (1999) Alcohol and injury: a comparison of emergency room populations in two Canadian provinces. Am J Drug Alcohol Abuse 25: 743–759

Chick J, Kreitman N, Plant M (1981) Mean cell volume and gamma-glutamyltranspeptidase as markers of drinking in working men. Lancet i: 1249–1251

Coccini T, Castoldi AF, Gandini C, Randine G, Vittadini G, Baiardi P, Manzo L (2002) Platelet monoamine oxidase B activity as a state marker for alcoholism: trend over time during withdrawal and influence of smoking and gender. Alcohol Alcohol 37: 566–572

Conigrave KM, Degenhardt LJ, Whitfield JB, Saunders JB, Helander A, Tabakoff B (2002) CDT, GGT, and AST as markers of alcohol use: the WHO/ISBRA collaborative project. Alcohol Clin Exp Res 26: 332–339

Dahl H, Stephanson N, Beck O, Helander A (2002) Comparison of urinary excretion characteristics of ethanol and ethyl glucuronide. J Anal Toxicol 26: 201–204

Davis VE, Brown H, Huff JA, Cashaw JL (1967) The alteration of serotonin metabolism to 5-hydroxytryptophol by ethanol ingestion in man. J Lab Clin Med 69: 132–140

DiMartini A, Day N, Lane T, Beisler AT, Dew MA, Anton R (2001) Carbohydrate deficient transferrin in abstaining patients with end-stage liver disease. Alcohol Clin Exp Res 25: 1729–1733

D'Onofrio G, Degutis LC (2002) Preventive care in the emergency department: screening and brief intervention for alcohol problems in the emergency department: a systematic review. Acad Emerg Med 9: 627–638

Dorafshar AH, O'Boyle DJ, McCloy RF (2002) Effects of a moderate dose of alcohol on simulated laparoscopic surgical performance. Surg Endosc 16: 1753–1758

Eggers V, Tio J, Neumann T, Pragst F, Muller C, Schmidt LG, Kox WJ, Spies CD (2002) Blood alcohol concentration for monitoring ethanol treatment to prevent alcohol withdrawal in the intensive care unit. Intensive Care Med 28: 1475–1482

Enoch MA, Goldman D (2001) The genetics of alcoholism and alcohol abuse. Curr Psychiatry Rep 3: 144–151

Freeze HH (2001) Update and perspectives on congenital disorders of glycosylation. Glycobiology 11: 129R–143R

Fuller RK, Lee KK, Gordis E (1988) Validity of self-report in alcoholism research: results of a Veterans Administration cooperative study. Alcohol Clin Exp Res 12: 201–205

Gelernter J, Goldman D, Risch N (1993) The A1 allele at the D2 dopamine receptor gene and alcoholism. A reappraisal. JAMA 269: 1673–1677

George S, Braithwaite RA (1995) An investigation into the extent of possible dilution of specimens received for urinary drugs of abuse screening. Addiction 90: 967–970

Hagan RL, Helander A (1997) Urinary 5-hydroxytryptophol following acute ethanol consumption: clinical evaluation and potential aviation applications. Aviat Space Environ Med 68: 30–34

Hearne R, Connolly A, Sheehan J (2002) Alcohol abuse: prevalence and detection in a general hospital. J R Soc Med 95: 84–87

Helander A (1999) Absolute or relative measurement of carbohydrate-deficient transferrin in serum? Experiences with three immunological assays. Clin Chem 45: 131–135

Helander A, Carlsson S (1996) Carbohydrate-deficient transferrin and gamma-glutamyl transferase levels during disulfiram therapy. Alcohol Clin Exp Res 20: 1202–1205

Helander A, Eriksson CJ (2002) Laboratory tests for acute alcohol consumption: results of the WHO/ISBRA Study on State and Trait Markers of Alcohol Use and Dependence. Alcohol Clin Exp Res 26: 1070–1077

Helander A, Beck O, Wennberg M, Wikström T, Jacobsson G (1991) Determination of urinary 5-hydroxyindole-3-acetic acid by high-performance liquid chromatography with electrochemical detection and direct sample injection. Anal Biochem 196: 170–173

Helander A, Wikström T, Löwenmo C, Jacobsson G, Beck O (1992) Urinary excretion of 5-hydroxyindole-3-acetic acid and 5-hydroxytryptophol after oral loading with serotonin. Life Sci 50: 1207–1213

Helander A, Beck O, Jacobsson G, Löwenmo C, Wikström T (1993) Time course of ethanol-induced changes in serotonin metabolism. Life Sci 53: 847–855

Helander A, Beck O, Jones AW (1995) Distinguishing ingested ethanol from microbial formation by analysis of urinary 5-hydroxytryptophol and 5-hydroxyindoleacetic acid. J Forens Sci 40: 95–98

Helander A, Beck O, Boysen L (1995) 5-Hydroxytryptophol conjugation in man: influence of alcohol consumption and altered serotonin turnover. Life Sci 56: 1529–1534

Helander A, Beck O, Jones AW (1996a) Laboratory testing for recent alcohol consumption: comparison of ethanol, methanol, and 5-hydroxytryptophol. Clin Chem 42: 618–624

Helander A, Voltaire Carlsson A, Borg S (1996b) Longitudinal comparison of carbohydrate-deficient transferrin and gamma-glutamyl transferase: complementary markers of excessive alcohol consumption. Alcohol Alcohol 31: 101–107

Helander A, von Wachenfeldt J, Hiltunen A, Beck O, Liljeberg P, Borg S (1999) Comparison of urinary 5-hydroxytryptophol, breath ethanol, and self- report for detection

of recent alcohol use during outpatient treatment: a study on methadone patients. Drug Alcohol Depend 56: 33–38
Helander A, Eriksson G, Stibler H, Jeppsson J-O (2001) Interference of transferrin isoform types with carbohydrate-deficient transferrin quantification in the identification of alcohol abuse. Clin Chem 47: 1225–1233
Hermansson U, Knutsson A, Rönnberg S, Brandt L (1998) Feasibility of brief intervention in the workplace for the detection and treatment of excessive alcohol consumption. Int J Occup Environ Health 4: 71–78
Hermansson U, Helander A, Huss A, Brandt L, Rönnberg S (2000) The Alcohol Use Disorders Identification Test (AUDIT) and carbohydrate-deficient transferrin (CDT) in a routine workplace health examination. Alcohol Clin Exp Res 24: 180–187
Higuchi S, Matsushita S, Murayama M, Takagi S, Hayashida M (1995) Alcohol and aldehyde dehydrogenase polymorphisms and the risk for alcoholism. Am J Psychiatry 152: 1219–1221
Hoffman PL, Glanz J, Tabakoff B (2002) Platelet adenylyl cyclase activity as a state or trait marker in alcohol dependence: results of the WHO/ISBRA Study on State and Trait Markers of Alcohol Use and Dependence. Alcohol Clin Exp Res 26: 1078–1087
Holt S, Stewart IC, Dixon JM, Elton RA, Taylor TV, Little K (1980) Alcohol and the emergency service patient. Br Med J 281: 638–640
Huseby NE, Bjordal E, Nilssen O, Barth T (1997) Utility of biological markers during outpatient treatment of alcohol-dependent subjects: carbohydrate-deficient transferrin responds to moderate changes in alcohol consumption. Alcohol Clin Exp Res 21: 1343–1346
Iffland R (1996) New ways to use biochemical indicators of alcohol abuse to regrant licences in a fairer manner after drunken driving in Germany. Alcohol Alcohol 31: 619–620
Irwin M, Baird S, Smith TL, Schuckit M (1988) Use of laboratory tests to monitor heavy drinking by alcoholic men discharged from a treatment program. Am J Psychiatry 145: 595–599
Jaakonmaki PI, Knox KL, Horning EC, Horning MG (1967) The characterization by gas-liquid chromatography of ethyl β-D-glucosiduronic acid as a metabolite of ethanol in rat and man. Eur J Pharmacol 1: 63–70
Jeppsson J-O, Kristensson H, Fimiani C (1993) Carbohydrate deficient transferrin quantitated by HPLC to determine heavy consumption of alcohol. Clin Chem 39: 2115–2120
Jones AW (1995) Measuring ethanol in saliva with the QED enzymatic test device: comparison of results with blood and breath-alcohol concentration. J Anal Toxicol 19: 169–173
Jones AW, Schuberth J (1989) Computer-aided headspace gas chromatography applied to blood-alcohol analysis: importance of on-line process control. J Forens Sci 34: 1116–1127
Jones AW, Helander A (1998) Changes in the concentrations of ethanol, methanol and metabolites of serotonin in two successive urinary voids from drinking drivers. Forensic Sci Int 93: 127–134
Jones AW, Hylén L, Svensson E, Helander A (1999) Storage of specimens at 4 degrees C or addition of sodium fluoride (1%) prevents formation of ethanol in urine inoculated with *Candida albicans*. J Anal Toxicol 23: 333–336
Kristenson H, Jeppsson J-O (1998) Drunken driver examinations. CD-transferrin is a valuable marker of alcohol consumption. Läkartidningen 95: 1429–1430
Kristenson H, Österling A, Nilsson JÅ, Lindgärde F (2002) Prevention of alcohol-related deaths in middle-aged heavy drinkers. Alcohol Clin Exp Res 26: 478–484
Landberg E, Påhlsson P, Lundblad A, Arnetorp A, Jeppsson J-O (1995) Carbohydrate composition of serum transferrin isoforms from patients with high alcohol consumption. Biochem Biophys Res Commun 210: 267–274

Martin MJ, Heymann C, Neumann T, Schmidt L, Soost F, Mazurek B, Bohm B, Marks C, Helling K, Lenzenhuber E, Muller C, Kox WJ, Spies CD (2002) Preoperative evaluation of chronic alcoholics assessed for surgery of the upper digestive tract. Alcohol Clin Exp Res 26: 836–840

McQuade WH, Levy SM, Yanek LR, Davis SW, Liepman MR (2000) Detecting symptoms of alcohol abuse in primary care settings. Arch Fam Med 9: 814–821

Meerkerk GJ, Njoo KH, Bongers IM, Trienekens P, van Oers JA (1998) The specificity of the CDT assay in general practice: the influence of common chronic diseases and medication on the serum CDT concentration. Alcohol Clin Exp Res 22: 908–913

Meerkerk GJ, Njoo KH, Bongers IM, Trienekens P, van Oers JA (1999) Comparing the diagnostic accuracy of carbohydrate-deficient transferrin, gamma-glutamyltransferase, and mean cell volume in a general practice population. Alcohol Clin Exp Res 23: 1052–1059

Midanik LT (1988) Validity of self-reported alcohol use: a literature review and assessment. Br J Addict 83: 1019–1030

Mitchell C, Simpson D, Chick J (1997) Carbohydrate deficient transferrin in detecting relapse in alcohol dependence. Drug Alcohol Depend 48: 97–103

Nilssen O, Førde OH (1994) Seven-year longitudinal population study of change in gamma-glutamyltransferase: the Tromsø study. Am J Epidemiol 139: 787–792

Nishikawa M, Tsuchihashi H, Miki A, Katagi M, Schmitt G, Zimmer H, Keller T, Aderjan R (1999) Determination of ethyl glucuronide, a minor metabolite of ethanol, in human serum by liquid chromatography-electrospray ionization mass spectrometry. J Chromatogr B Biomed Sci Appl 726: 105–110

Peter J, Unverzagt C, Engel WD, Renauer D, Seidel C, Hosel W (1998) Identification of carbohydrate deficient transferrin forms by MALDI-TOF mass spectrometry and lectin ELISA. Biochim Biophys Acta 1380: 93–101

Ragland DR, Krause N, Greiner BA, Holman BL, Fisher JM, Cunradi CB (2002) Alcohol consumption and incidence of workers' compensation claims: a 5-year prospective study of urban transit operators. Alcohol Clin Exp Res 26: 1388–1394

Ratsma JE, Van Der Stelt O, Gunning WB (2002) Neurochemical markers of alcoholism vulnerability in humans. Alcohol Alcohol 37: 522–533

Reid MC, Fiellin DA, O'Connor PG (1999) Hazardous and harmful alcohol consumption in primary care. Arch Intern Med 159: 1681–1689

Rosalki SB, Rau D (1972) Serum gamma-glutamyl transpeptidase activity in alcoholism. Clin Chim Acta 39: 41–47

Rosman AS, Basu P, Galvin K, Lieber CS (1995) Utility of carbohydrate-deficient transferrin as a marker of relapse in alcoholic patients. Alcohol Clin Exp Res 19: 611–616

Schmitt G, Aderjan R, Keller T, Wu M (1995) Ethyl glucuronide: an unusual ethanol metabolite in humans. Synthesis, analytical data, and determination in serum and urine. J Anal Toxicol 19: 91–94

Schmitt G, Droenner P, Skopp G, Aderjan R (1997) Ethyl glucuronide concentration in serum of human volunteers, teetotalers, and suspected drinking drivers. J Forensic Sci 42: 1099–1102

Schuckit MA (2000) Genetics of the risk for alcoholism. Am J Addict 9: 103–112

Seidl S, Wurst FM, Alt A (2001) Ethyl glucuronide — a biological marker for recent alcohol consumption. Addict Biol 6: 205–212

Shepherd J (1994) Violent crime: the role of alcohol and new approaches to the prevention of injury. Alcohol Alcohol 29: 5–10

Smolle KH, Hofmann G, Kaufmann P, Lueger A, Brunner G (1999) Q.E.D. Alcohol test: a simple and quick method to detect ethanol in saliva of patients in emergency departments. Comparison with the conventional determination in blood. Intensive Care Med 25: 492–495

Spies CD, Nordmann A, Brummer G, Marks C, Conrad C, Berger G, Runkel N, Neumann T, Müller C, Rommelspacher H, Specht M, Hannemann L, Striebel HW, Schaffartzik W (1996) Intensive care unit stay is prolonged in chronic alcoholic men following tumor resection of the upper digestive tract. Acta Anaesthesiol Scand 40: 649–656

Spies CD, Kissner M, Neumann T, Blum S, Voigt C, Funk T, Runkel N, Pragst F (1998) Elevated carbohydrate-deficient transferrin predicts prolonged intensive care unit stay in traumatized men. Alcohol Alcohol 33: 661–669

Spies CD, Herpell J, Beck O, Muller C, Pragst F, Borg S, Helander A (1999) The urinary ratio of 5-hydroxytryptophol to 5-hydroxyindole-3-acetic acid in surgical patients with chronic alcohol misuse. Alcohol 17: 19–27

Staak M, Iffland R (1992) Alcoholism detection markers in blood samples of road users. Arukoru Kenkyuto Yakubutsu Izon 27: 42–49

Stephanson N, Dahl H, Helander A, Beck O (2002) Direct quantification of ethyl glucuronide in clinical urine samples by liquid chromatography-mass spectrometry. Ther Drug Monit 24: 645–651

Stibler H (1991) Carbohydrate-deficient transferrin in serum: a new marker of potentially harmful alcohol consumption reviewed. Clin Chem 37: 2029–2037

Svensson S, Some M, Lundsjö A, Helander A, Cronholm T, Höög J-O (1999) Activities of human alcohol dehydrogenases in the metabolic pathways of ethanol and serotonin. Eur J Biochem 262: 324–329

Tanaka K, Tokunaga S, Kono S, Tokudome S, Akamatsu T, Moriyama T, Zakouji H (1998) Coffee consumption and decreased serum gamma-glutamyltransferase and aminotransferase activities among male alcohol drinkers. Int J Epidemiol 27: 438–443

Tønnesen H (1999) The alcohol patient and surgery. Alcohol Alcohol 34: 148–152

Tønnesen H, Carstensen M, Maina P (1999) Is carbohydrate deficient transferrin a useful marker of harmful alcohol intake among surgical patients? Eur J Surg 165: 522–527

Voltaire A, Beck O, Borg S (1992) Urinary 5-hydroxytryptophol: a possible marker of recent alcohol consumption. Alcohol Clin Exp Res 16: 281–285

Voltaire Carlsson A, Hiltunen AJ, Beck O, Stibler H, Borg S (1993) Detection of relapses in alcohol-dependent patients: comparison of carbohydrate-deficient transferrin in serum, 5-hydroxytryptophol in urine, and self-reports. Alcohol Clin Exp Res 17: 703–708

Wiese JG, Shlipak MG, Browner WS (2000) The alcohol hangover. Ann Intern Med 132: 897–902

Yesavage JA, Dolhert N, Taylor JL (1994) Flight simulator performance of younger and older aircraft pilots: effects of age and alcohol. J Am Geriatr Soc 42: 577–582

Yokoyama A, Muramatsu T, Omori T, Yokoyama T, Matsushita S, Higuchi S, Maruyama K, Ishii H (2001) Alcohol and aldehyde dehydrogenase gene polymorphisms and oropharyngolaryngeal, esophageal and stomach cancers in Japanese alcoholics. Carcinogenesis 22: 433–439

Zweig MH, Campbell G (1993) Receiver-operating characteristic (ROC) plots: a fundamental evaluation tool in clinical medicine. Clin Chem 39: 561–577

Author's address: Dr. A. Helander, Alcohol Laboratory, L7:03, Karolinska Hospital, SE-171 76 Stockholm, Sweden, e-mail: anders.helander@cns.ki.se

Substitution management in opioid dependence

A. Uchtenhagen

Addiction Research Institute, Zurich, Switzerland

Summary. Substitution treatment (replacement therapy) is the most widespread and the most frequently researched therapeutic approach to heroin dependence. At present, the "gold standard" is methadone maintenance, but the use of other agonists and of combined compounds with antagonists are increasingly used, especially Buprenorphine. This paper reviews the main findings from research and their consequences for best practice rules. The evolution and organisation of substitution treatment in Europe is described, indicating a major discrepancy in administrative regulations. Emerging trends are also mentioned, as well as the merits and limitations that mark the place of substitution treatment in a comprehensive therapeutic network for opioid dependence.

Definition and objectives

Substitution treatment is a therapeutic option that includes the prescription of agonist substances as an adjunct to medical and psychosocial care. The indication and the duration of treatment are determined on the basis of an individual assessment.

Substitution treatment is at present available for opiate dependent persons only. As a rule the opiate of abuse is diacetylmorphine (Heroin). Earlier prescription of alcohol to alcohol dependent persons has been proven to be ineffective and was abandoned. Medical prescription of stimulants as a substitution treatment is sporadically practised, not adequately evaluated and controversial.

The objectives of prescribing opoid agonists as a substitution for heroin are the following:

- to replace the unhygienic, uncontrolled and risky forms of illegal heroin administration (especially intravenous injections)
- to reduce all activities linked to the purchase of illegal heroin
- to facilitate a reorientation of heroin dependent persons towards a socially integrated, healthy, responsible life-style
- to improve the chances for a final abstinence from opiates.

The objectives of substitution treatment do not diverge essentially from those of abstinence-oriented treatment. However, there is a difference regarding the timing of intermediate objectives: while abstinence-oriented treatments regard abstinence as a prerequisite for better health and social status (and therefore prefer residential settings), substitution treatment attempts to improve health and social status in order to better achieve permanent abstinence (and consequently prefers out-patient settings). Substitution treatment also allows to reach intermediate goals where the ultimate objective of abstinence cannot be reached yet or at all, as a palliative treatment or as a risk reducing measure.

Pharmacological basis

The substitution of diacetylmorphine by opioid agonists is based on their affinity to μ-δ- and κ-receptors. This is the case for morphine, methadone, levo-alpha-acetylmethadol LAAM, and also for mono-acetylmorphine, a metabolite of diamorphine. Buprenorphine and, to a lesser degree, Codeine also bind to μ-receptors. When these receptors are taken by substitution agonists, no withdrawal symptoms may develop and additional heroin cannot become effective.

When opioids are continuously administered, a combination of mechanisms induces tolerance; higher dosages are needed for having the same effects. At the same time, higher dosages can be tolerated which might be lethal in non-tolerant individuals. There is cross-tolerance between the abovementioned opioids. Prescribed opioids induce tolerance for the effects of heroin. Discontinuation of substitution is followed by a withdrawal state comparable to the state after cessation of heroin administration, and tolerance is gradually diminishing. After complete withdrawal the same lethal dosages apply as in non-tolerant individuals.

Not all opioids have exactly the same effects. For substitution purposes the following are relevant: longer duration of action in comparison to heroin, less euphoria producing, oral applicability. These characteristics made the synthetic compound Methadone the preferred substitution opioid. Today the main emphasis is to determine which agonist is preferable under the specific circumstances of each patient.

Indication

Substitution treatment was considered to be a treatment of second choice, if abstinence oriented treatment was not available, not feasible, or had repeatedly failed. When Dole and Nyswander introduced Methadone substitution in 1965, they set up strict entry criteria: minimal age of 21 years, minimal duration of heroin dependence of 4 years, no serious psychopathology, no problems with alcohol or other substances of abuse, multiple failures in other treatment approaches. As polydrug use and polydrug dependence became more frequent, it was unrealistic to exclude them from substitution treatment. The HIV epidemic, the rapid increase of AIDS cases in drug injectors and a transmission of HIV infections to their sexual partners signaled such a threat to public health that substitution treatment became an option to reduce such risks and the access to treatment was facilitated.

At present the following general rules apply for the indication:

— confirmed opiate dependence (following the criteria of ICD-10 or DSM-IV)
— informed consent to accept the conditions of substitution treatment
— no contraindication.

Further conditions have to be considered:

— detailed history (biography, health and social history, history of addictive behavior including consumption patterns, consequences of substance use, former treatment attempts etc)
— present living situation (housing, occupation, income, network, perspectives)
— complementary medical and/or psychiatric examination regarding indicators for a comorbidity (not in order to exclude such patients, but in the interest of a comprehensive treatment planning)
— extensive information on all available treatment options, and advise on the most appropriate option for the situation and the problem at stake
— shared identification of treatment goals (detoxification, interim substitution, mid- or long-term substitution)
— identification of the most appropriate substitution medication
— discussion and identification of the conditions and modalities, preferably using a written informed consent statement.

Detoxification using substitution medication with a reduction scheme releaves withdrawal symptoms, but eventually prolongs the withdrawal syndrome (especially when using long-acting medications such as methadone).

Interim substitution and other forms of short-term substitution treatment may be helpful in specific situations, such as pregnancy, urgent hospitalization (which would not be accepted without substitution), physical conditions necessitating an interruption of risky injections. The duration of interim substitution is determined on the nature of the specific situation.

Long-term substitution is to be considered if opiate dependence is already chronic and if an abstinence-oriented treatment is not accepted (e.g. in order not to loose a job or because a somatic or psychiatric condition impede participation in a residential program).

General normative conditions such as minimal age, duration of dependence, number of previous treatments that failed are not to be recommended. However, substitution treatment must be carefully weighed if dependence is a recent development, especially in minors.

The duration of long-term substitution should not be limited administratively. Routine limitation not respecting the individual situation increases the risk for relapse after the termination of treatment (Ward et al., 1998).

Substitution treatment is *not an emergency treatment*, with the exception of some physical conditions like *morbus embolicus* or myocardial infection. On the other side, the assessment should not take too much time, in order not to spoil a positive motivation for treatment. It has been evidenced that within 2 weeks on a waiting list many patients already get lost, and not necessarily those with a poor prognosis (Maddux et al., 1995).

When the initial prognosis for the feasibility of a substitution treatment is unclear, the indication may be limited to a *trial period*, delaying the definite indication for e.g. 3 months. It is recommended to reconsider the indication periodically, at least every 2 years.

The indication for a substitution treatment should be made by a physician who has adequate experience in the management of heroin dependents, who knows abstinence oriented treatment as well as substitution treatment. In some countries the right to determine the indication is reserved to physicians with adequate experience or who accept continued education on the problems and modalities of addiction treatment.

Absolute contraindications are not known (except failing opiate dependence).

Relative contradindications are: acute hepatic conditions, severe hepatic insufficiency (risk of overdose from retarded metabolisation), respiratory deficiency (risk of oxygen deficit due to respiratory depression from opioids), individual oversensitivity to a specific opioid, age under 18 years. A partial detoxification is recommended previous to starting substitution treatment in the presence of a dependence from alcohol or Benzodiazepines (risk of a respiratory deficiency due to combined action). Psychotic and otherwise mentally impaired patients (e.g. patients with AIDS encephalitis) will need careful assessment with regard to their coping ability for a substitution treatment, eventually in collaboration with relatives or other key persons.

Pregnancy is no contraindication for a substitution treatment.

Implementation

The care programme

Ancillary care is of utmost importance for the outcome of substitution treatment. It must be tailored to the individual needs of the patient. Comparative analysis of Methadone programs has demonstrated that a comprehensive care program allows for better retention rates and better outcome (Ball and Ross, 1991; McLellan et al., 1993). A care program respecting the needs for medical treatment and for social and rehabilitative measures is equally important as the prescription of a substitution medication. Clearly formulated agreements between doctor and patient help to prevent and to manage problematic situations. Such an agreement should eventually include other concerned parties (psychotherapist, social worker, pharmacist, parole officer, partner).

Psychosocial care includes advise in financial and juridical matters, in job placement or job seeking, in housing problems, in all kinds of crisis situations. It includes advise for spouses or relatives, and the provision of contact with other agencies. Psychosocial care must adapt to changing situations in the course of treatment. The same holds for the frequency of consultations: initially and in crisis more frequent and more intensive consultation is needed. Consultation mainly focuses on improving living conditions and life-style, provides therapeutic support and monitors the status in physical and psychological health.

Psychotherapy may support the treatment process considerably. A specific indication is needed however, considering the individual condition and also the suitability for a psychotherapeutic method, be it an individual or a systemic treatment. When carefully indicated, psychotherapy may improve the outcome of a substitution treatment (Woody, 1995). Group therapy is an integrated element in many substitution treatment programs; the need for an individual indication is less important than the need to assess eventual contraindications (e.g. in psychotic or severely depressive patients).

Good psychosocial care asks for professional competence in various fields. It is therefore often provided on an *interdisciplinary basis*, in a multiprofessional team or in collaboration between physician and a specialized consultation agency. The medical responsibility is with the prescribing physician. A coordination of the various care elements by case management is recommended.

Psychosocial care must also consider the patient's motivation for treatment and readiness for change. Forced consultations may lead to breaking off treatment completely, especially when the patient is healthy and well integrated, and sees no reason for regular intensive care. Indeed, substitution treatment in well integrated patients was found to reduce illegal drug consumption and its risks also without much ancillary care (Raschke et al., 1994). On the other side, many patients need *motivational support* in order to accept treatment and care. Motivation techniques have been developed and implemented primarily in the US (Simpson et al., 1997). Examples are reward systems (bonuses, reduction of controls, take-home privileges for Methadone) for compliant behavior such as regular participation in group meetings and individual consultation sessions (Chutuape, 1998). Another technique focuses on enhancing problem awareness by linking individual problems to addictive behavior (node-link mapping technique, Dees, 1997).

Some experiments with *low-threshold Methadone prescription* in the Netherlands and in Switzerland have demonstrated the feasibility of a safe prescription practice without ancillary psychosocial care, if controlled daily Methadone intake is provided and measures against overdosing are taken. When offered to heroin dependents who are reluctant to engage in a care program, results seem to be doubtful, although transition to a well structured Methadone program is encouraged. Also, a reduction of infection risks in a low-threshold regime could not be evidenced (Ward et al., 1998). The regime seems to be better justified in cases without major health or social deficits. There are no studies on the mid- and long-term outcome at present.

Management and treatment of comorbidity

Conditions that preceded drug dependence or emerged as their consequence must be assessed *lege artis* in order to receive adequate treatment by the prescribing physician or in collaboration with a specialist or with the family doctor of the patient. Two problem areas have to be kept in mind:

- — interactions between substitution medication and other medications
- — interference between the various therapeutic regimes if those are not clearly defined and coordinated, leading to irritations and inviting manipulative behavior.

Main somatic conditions associated to heroin dependence are a range of infectious diseases, malnutrition, caries etc. When adequately treated during a substitution regime they may improve rather quickly, due to the discontinuation of risky injections and an improvement of living conditions. The immune system is improving, and the risk for an HIV- or Hepatitis infection is diminishing (Ward et al., 1998).

Interactions of medications must be considered. For instance, tuberculostatic drugs such as Rifamcipin and Rifabutin, antiepileptic drugs like Phenytoin as well as some barbiturates and Benzodiazepines enhance the metabolisation of Methadone by enzyme induction (P450 oxydase system). This may be compensated by increasing the frequency of oral Methadone intake, not by increasing the dosage. On the other side, Chinidin, Clozapin, Betablockers and Antiarrhythmica may impede metabolisation through competitive inhibition, such increasing the risk for overdosing (overview see Ward et al., 1998).

Psychiatric conditions associated to Heroin dependence (dual diagnoses) are depressive disorders, anxiety disorders, post-traumatic stress syndrome, personality disorders and schizophrenic psychosis (ranged according to frequency of prevalence). They may be a consequence of dependence; if preceding dependence, Heroin use may be understood as a form of self-medication. Stress may be an underlying factor contributing to both Heroin use and the psychiatric disorder. The psychiatric symptoms can be improved in the course of a substitution treatment, especially if the addictive behavior has contributed to its manifestation. Often however they need to be treated according to the specific diagnosis. It is recommended to reassess the psychological status when the Methadone dosage has been stabilised; if psychiatric symptoms are persisting, a specific treatment has to be started (Ward et al., 1998). Patients with schizophrenic symptoms need a well structured regime without the confrontations often used in the treatment of substance dependence, and an antipsychotic medication. There are no general rules for the management of opiate dependents with personality disorders; a good therapeutic climate and well trained therapists will be essential.

Regarding interactions, the competitive inhibition of Methadone metabolisation by tricyclic and tetracyclic antidepressants, by fluvoxamine, by serotinin reuptake inhibitors and some neuroleptics are to be respected (Ward et al., 1998; Bertschy, 1995).

Polydrug dependence

Simultaneous dependence from more than one substance of abuse is a major impediment for a successful substitution treatment. It is an obstacle against positive changes in life-style, and it increases risks, e.g. for respiratory depression, on the basis of synergic pharmacological action. Mortality during Methadone substitution treatment is mainly due to an additional intake of alcohol, barbiturates or Benzodiazepines. The risk for a Hepatitis or HIV infection is increased in patients with an additional dependence on Cocaine (especially if Cocaine is injected, but also if Crack is used in conjunction with unsafe sex practices). Continued contact with the illegal drug market with ensuing temptations and risks is another negative consequence of Cocaine dependence.

Polydrug use is frequently reduced in Methadone substitution treatment, if dosage and psychosocial care are adequate. This effect may be enhanced through behavioral therapy measures (bonuses for "clean urines", reversal of privileges after "dirty urines"). Polydrug dependence may ask for additional measures. Partial detoxification treatment or drug specific combination treatments are recommended. Sanctions however, especially exclusion from treatment after a given number of positive urines increase the risks for relapse and mortality and are not recommended (Wrad et al., 1998).

A regime used for a reduction of Cocaine consumption is an antidepressant medication, especially in the presence of depressive symptoms. Positive outcome was reported when prescribing Imipramin, while controlled studies with Desipramin, Amantadin and Bromocriptin had no effect on Cocaine use (overview by Mattick et al., 1998). Anticraving medication (Acamprosat) has not been systematically tested yet for its efficacy against Cocaine use. Psychotherapy using contingency contracting has also been applied with contradictory results.

Alcohol dependence in opiate addicts has attracted less attention by therapists and researchers in comparison to Cocaine dependence. Alcohol dependence however has a major role in making a Methadone regime difficult, and it increases the mortality risk in treated and untreated Heroin dependence. It may persist even in cases of successfully treated Heroin dependence and increase the risk for later relapse. All therapeutic measures developed for the treatment of alcohol dependence and for hazardous alcohol use can be applied during Methadone substitution treatment. This includes out-patient early intervention techniques, aversive therapies, participation in self-help groups and other relapse prevention methods. Disulfiram as an aversive medication shortens the metabolisation of Methadone and invites a higher frequency of intake.

Benzodiazepine dependence and dependence from other sedatives is a frequent and serious complication in Heroin addicts. Most prevalent is the use of Flunitrazepam. An avoidable reason for using it is an insufficient dosage of Methadone.

Control measures

An essential element, especially during the starting phase and crisis periods, eventually during the entire treatment, is the visually *controlled intake* of Methadone. The daily controlled intake must be combined with the control of a special permit in a Methadone program where the number of patients excludes a reliable identification of each individual person. Controlled intake may not be feasible where the service or the pharmacy is closed on weekends; in this case, one or two daily doses have to be taken home on Fridays.

In a later stage, when dosages and the living conditions of a patient have become stable, a *take-home policy* for a couple of days may be applied.

Take-home and frequency of consultations are not following uniform rules; they depend on the attitude and the experience of the prescribing physician, on official regulations and local traditions. The advantages of a take-home policy include a better retention of patients who have become stable (Rhoades et al., 1998) and a better compliance (Stitzer et al., 1992). It also facilitates the vocational rehabilitation of patients.

Disadvantages are the additional risks for patients who are not sufficiently stable, as they may loose or sell their Methadone and replace it by illegal injections, or they may use more than one daily dose at once. Especially the mortality risk is increased in such cases, due to overdosing of patients or of other persons who have no opiate tolerance. Also, prescribed Methadone may be found on the illegal market and lead to discredit of substitution treatment. All these disadvantages and risks can be avoided, if take-home is granted to patients only who are stable enough (Senay et al., 1994).

Take away doses of Methadone should not replaced if claimed to be lost. Administration through third parties is not recommended, with the exception of reliable relatives or other key persons well known to the prescribing physician, and only if the patient is physically unable to visit the Methadone clinic regularly.

Urine controls are traditionally another essential element of a Methadone program. In many instances they are officially requested, in some countries they are merely recommended. Urine controls are made without previous announcement. Visual control, temperature control or testing for substances added to the oral Methadone suspension are practiced in order to recognize a urine which was brought in. The rationale for urine controls is the recognition of non-prescribed substances and an evidence for the intake of prescribed Methadone.

The high costs of urine controls and a dislike by staff and patients for this kind of control have invited research on the usefulness of such measures. It has been evidenced that frequent and regular controls are not necessary. Infrequent and irregular controls are not linked to an increase in illegal drug use or to less favorable outcomes (Ward et al., 1998).

In everyday practice, urine controls still have a role. The frequency is highly variable. It is not recommended to leave out controls completely, even in cases of good compliance, because an objectively established drug-free status may reinforce considerably the patient's self-esteem and self-control.

Frequent controls are made in the initial treatment phase and in crisis situations.

Analysis is usually made for heroin and other opioids, eventually also for Benzodiazepines, barbiturates and Cocaine.

If illegal or non-prescribed substances are detected, this must be openly discussed with the patient. Circumstances connected to the use of such substances, ensuing risks, motivation for a better compliance, and measures to be expected if noncompliant behavior continues are the main topics for discussion. The results have to be documented in the case history. Without this process, urine controls have little value.

Urine controls are also used for documenting the evolution of the patient's behavior, for administrative or legal purposes, e.g. in order to obtain a drivers license. Informed consent with passing relevant information to the authorities concerned must be assured.

Duration and termination of treatment

The duration of substitution treatments must be determined for each patient individually. Rigid and schematic limitations of the duration are counterproductive and increase the relapse risk (Caplehorn, 1994).

Improvement in health status, reduction of illegal Heroin use and of Heroin-related delinquency are observed within months. It takes more time to build up new social contacts and to become reintegrated into the labor market. One to two years are usually needed in order to reach a stable consolidation of living conditions and durable behavior change. In many instances further improvements are still made after a couple of years. However, after three to four years the chances for improvements tend to become lower, and there may be a risk for secondary deterioration and resignation.

Many patients are impatient and ask for an early termination of substitution treatment. They want to prove, to themselves and to others, that they are perfectly well prepared for a drug-free life. It is an essential therapeutic task to motivate these patients for a prolonged treatment and a stepwise procedure, comparable to what is needed for a prolonged antipsychotic medication for schizophrenia or an aversive treatment with Disulfiram for alcohol dependence. Less experienced doctors often consider a short substitution treatment to be preferable, unaware of the risks for relapse after a short treatment and of a negative effect on the motivation to take up treatment again if it failed. On the other side, there are patients who cannot find the courage to terminate substitution treatment after years of a satisfactory consolidation and reintegration. Those may need encouragement to engage in a stepwise termination. And again, there are other patients who are unable to "mature-out" or "age-out" of a dependence-prone state of mind and who may need substitution treatment for many years. The basis for such a condition has not been clarified yet.

The termination of treatment must be well prepared with clearly defined steps, together with the patient. This includes timing and extent of dose reductions, modality of final detoxification, continued after-care, management of later crisis situations, and options for restarting substitution treatment if needed.

It is recommended to break off treatment if the patient continuously does not comply with what had been agreed upon, if he takes Methadone on an irregular basis only, if he behaves aggressively towards staff, if he is selling prescribed substances or engages otherwise in drug trafficking. Continued consumption of non-prescribed drugs is a reason for breaking-off if there is a vital risk for overdosing. In any case, a careful consideration of the risks from keeping the patient in treatment against breaking off treatment should guide such a far-reaching decision.

Whenever and however a substitution treatment is terminated, care should be taken to keep options open for returning to treatment, in the same program or in another service. Coming back to treatment should not be prohibitively labeled as a failure for the patient or for the therapist. It has been shown that returning to treatment is a real chance and may lead to better results.

Special problems

Substitution treatment and driving

The ability and permission to drive a motor vehicle is of importance for practical reasons and especially for vocational rehabilitation. Many patients have lost their driver's license on the basis of their Heroin dependence. In order to regain the license, they must present no unusual risks to road safety. Such unusual risks can be excluded on the basis of an assessment of the health status, of documented drug-free urines over a defined period of time and of the patient's general behavior. Assessment is made independently, not by the prescribing physician, but the responsible agency as a rule consults him for his observations and prognosis.

The individual assessment of the patient's driving ability does not use uniform criteria. As a rule, a minimal duration of 6 to 12 months on substitution with stable dosage is required. Other requirements are an adequate status in somatic and psychological health, a stable housing condition, absence of delinquent and otherwise irresponsible behavior, and abstinence from illegal and non-prescribed substances (documented through urine analysis).

Driving ability is not per se impaired by substitution medication, if dosage is stable and full opiate tolerance is reached, and if intake is regular. In the case of oral Methadone it is evidenced that attention, coordination and reactivity are but minimally impaired under steady-state conditions (Seidenberg and Honegger, 1998). The use of short-acting substitution drugs is more problematic.

Overdosing in substitution medication may lead to impaired driving if opiate tolerance is not fully developed. Underdosing on the other side invites collateral use of other substances that may have a negative impact on driving.

In case of relapse into illegal or non-prescribed substance use, the treating physician must determine if his patient is still able to drive or if he has to report the patient's inability to the authority concerned.

Substitution treatment during vacations

Mainstream lifestyle includes the possibilities to go some place for a holiday. Social integration and engaging in social relations with friends and partners is made difficult if you are not allowed to move to a holiday resort or to another country. The wish to go for a holiday therefore is often coming up during substitution treatment. The treating physician must decide whether it is acceptable to hand out substitution drugs in the amounts needed for a vacation, on the basis of the individual circumstances (stabilisation of dosage and living circumstances, reliability of patient, duration of vacation).

In many places and countries it is possible to arrange for a controlled intake of substitution drugs, but the options have to be explored and there may be some administrative problems to be dealt with. The respective national laws and regulations must be respected, and the availability of the drug must be checked. As a rule, in countries where Methadone substitution treatment is an accepted therapeutic modality, such an arrangement can be made. A medical certificate confirming the substitution treatment of the patient can be useful. It is not recommended to take the drugs into another country; being found out at border control may provoke serious problems.

Substitution treatment in prison

In most countries where Heroin dependence is a problem there are major difficulties in the prison milieu, for dependent inmates as well as for the institutions and their staff. One difficulty concerns the withdrawal syndromes of newly admitted dependents. Another frequent difficulty is the continued opiate use while being imprisoned, which presents specific health problems on the basis of needle and syringe sharing leading to blood-borne infections with HIV and hepatitis. Still another difficulty are the occasional overdose deaths.

In some countries an ongoing substitution treatment can be continued after imprisonment, in some others such a treatment can even be started while being in prison. More widespread is the practice of using Methadone in the detoxification of inmates (Dolan et al., 1998). Substitution treatment is practised as a special regime for some individuals, or else in special units. In any case such a treatment should be voluntary. Ideally inmates should be able to opt between a substitution treatment and a drug-free treatment. Evaluation of such practices is not adequately developed so far.

While being on remand, withdrawal symptoms may impair the prisoner's fitness for examination. This is not the case if the prisoner is under substitution treatment with adequate doses; the suicide risk is also reduced.

Ideally a substitution treatment in prison should be based on consultation with an external specialised agency which has already treated the patient or is going to take over after his release. Organising proper after-care is essential in preventing relapse.

Substitution treatment in hospital

An ongoing substitution treatment should be continued in case of temporary hospitalisation, be it in a somatic or a psychiatric hospital, if there are no medical contra-indications. If this is not provided, many patients in need of hospital treatment do not agree to be hospitalised or leave the hospital before treatment of their illness has a chance to improve their situation.

Also, the indication for starting a substitution treatment should be made if a hospitalisation is otherwise not feasible. Hospital physicians must be competent for such an indication, and clear rules on the regime must exist which are known to staff and to the respective patient. Successful substitution treatment is enhanced if good contact is established with external agencies that have already treated the patient or will be engaged in his after-care.

Substitution treatment during pregnancy

Patient's health status often improves considerably in the course of substitution treatments. Women patients restart to menstruate within months. If not adequately instructed or willing to use contraceptive measures they may become pregnant unintentionally, as they did not become pregnant while being on illegal drugs even without contraceptive measures.

In case of pregnancy the following options must be considered:

— If the woman wants to terminate substitution treatment the risks of withdrawal syndromes must be discussed, as spontaneous abortion may occur (Finnegan et al., 1991). In any case the dosages have to be carefully reduced, preferably between the weeks 14 and 32 in order to avoid abortion or premature delivery (Ward et al., 1998). It is contraindicated to use Benzodiazepines in order to avoid withdrawal symptoms. There is also a major risk for relapse into illegal heroin use after detoxification (Finnegan et al., 1991), and retention in a follow-up drug-free treatment is much lower than in substitution (Svikis et al., 1997).

— If the woman decides to continue substitution treatment, the advantages and potential disadvantages must also be considered. Methadone has less risks for the child in terms of birth weight and chromosome damage, in comparison with illegal heroin (Finnegan et al., 1991). A disadvantage is the withdrawal syndrome in the newborn child, and especially the risks for mid- and long-term effects on the child's development — risks which are not sufficiently explored yet. Neuro-psychological impairments and the respective behaviour disorders cannot be excluded, although milieu factors such as lifestyle and living conditions of the mother seem to have more impact on development than pharmacological factors (Lifschitz et al., 1985). It is important to notice that doses of Methadone should not be minimal but sufficient in order to prevent withdrawal symptoms and thereby collateral illegal or non-prescribed use of drugs. It is recommended to split daily doses in two to be taken with an appropriate interval in order to facilitate continued blood levels and to avoid peak concentrations. After childbirth Methadone substitution is compatible with breast-feeding; problems arise only in cases of harmful use of alcohol or other drugs.

Experience with and scientific evidence on the potential of other substitution drugs than Methadone is still insufficient.

The conclusion is that continuing Methadone substitution during pregnancy has more advantages than disadvantages, but those have to be checked in each individual case. However, such a conclusion can only be made for a qualified substitution treatment and under the condition that there is no parallel use of illegal heroin. The situation must be examined in a similar fashion if a pregnant woman applies for Methadone substitution treatment. The main reasons for starting substitution during pregnancy are avoiding the risks of illegal heroin use and the chances for guidance and consultation during pregnancy and childbed.

Substances used in opiate substitution

In some Asian countries (Laos, Pakistan) where opium used to be an important substance for medical and leisure purposes, opium was made available for dependent persons, though not in a therapeutic framework. These systems were abolished following the Single Convention of 1961 and under international pressure.

At present the following substances are prescribed as substitutes for heroin:

— Methadone (oral, intravenous)
— Levo-alpha-acetylmethadol LAAM (oral)
— Morphine (oral, intramuscular, intravenous)
— Codeine, Dihydrocodeine (oral)
— Buprenorphine (oral, intramuscular, intravenous)
— Diacetylmorphine (Heroin) (oral, intravenous).

Methadone

Oral Methadone is by far the most frequently used substance in opiate substitution treatment. It is mostly applied as a mixture of the pharmacologically active l-form and the inactive r-form. Research also has mostly focused on this modality. Preparations containing only the l-form were used especially in Germany but are increasingly replaced. Intravenous application is traditionally a therapeutic option in England where it is still an accepted modality (Metrebian et al., 1998). This modality was also tested in a Swiss study and found little acceptance, due to frequent and severe side-effects on the basis of comparatively high doses (Uchtenhagen et al., 1999).

The following statements concern the oral application. Oral Methadone has a bioavailability of 90–100%.

Initial doses correspond to the extent of opiate tolerance in a given patient. They are to be handled cautiously in order to avoid overdose. If tolerance is not clearly evident, doses should not exceed 30 mg/day, in cases of evident tolerance 60 mg/day split in two partial doses should not be exceeded. Increasing of doses is following observations on withdrawal symptoms. It is advisable to see the patient once or twice a day in order to prevent unpredictable complications. Only exceptionally it is necessary to hospitalise a patient for determining the adequate dosage.

Maintenance doses must be individually determined. The recommended medium range is between 60 and 100 mg per day. The maximum dosages formulated for non-tolerant persons do not apply. The general rule is not to prescribe minimal or maximal doses but doses that are sufficient in order to avoid withdrawal symptoms. Randomised trials have demonstrated that low doses around 30 mg per day are more frequently followed by dropping out of treatment, by collateral use of illegal substances and by less favourable outcomes, in comparison to dosages around 80 mg per day (overview by Ward et al., 1998). On the other side, an individually inappropriate high dosage may also invite non-prescribed Benzodiazepine or illegal cocaine use. If daily intake is interrupted, the dose has to be reduced in order to avoid overdose; per each day with missing Methadone intake it is recommended to reduce the dose by 20% (Seidenberg and Honegger, 1998).

There are no strict correlations found between dosage, plasma level and treatment outcome. It must be noted however that plasma levels and pharmacological action can be influenced by intervening illness and by interactions with other medications (see paragraph on the treatment of comorbidity). This may invite adjustments of dosage. Also it must be remembered that there are persons who metabolise Methadone quicker than the average and who therefore need higher doses.

Dose reduction before ending treatment is recommended, with a weekly reduction of the daily dose by 5–10 mg. The final reduction may use even smaller steps or else is made in a residential facility in order to avoid an early relapse. Many patients would prefer a quicker reduction, but in order to avoid relapse the individual reasons for doing so must be well examined.

The most frequent clinical *side-effects* of Methadone are constipation, sweating, sleep disorders and a reduced sexual appetite (libido). They can often be managed by dose adjustments and only rarely lead to a premature termination of treatment. Side-effects which are detected only in laboratory testing are clinically barely relevant (overview by Seidenberg and Honegger, 1998). A comprehensive presentation of the pharmacological and toxicological aspects is provided in Cooper et al. (1983).

Death during Methadone treatment occurs in the initial phase if there is no sufficient tolerance or if initial doses are too high. Death in the course of treatment is mostly due to a combination of Methadone and other substances (Benzodiazepines, barbiturates, alcohol), while Methadone only is rarely found in autopsies of overdose deaths (Ward et al., 1998; Scott et al., 1999).

LAAM (Levo-alpha.acetylmethadol)

LAAM has been developed for a long-term substitution treatment of patients with stable doses, on the basis of its longer half-life (2.6 days, active metabolites up to 4 days). Intake frequency can be reduced to 3 times a week with a dose of 100 mg each time. This is expected to have practical advantages, and the patients are less limited in their mobility.

On the other side, the longer duration of pharmacological action also means less flexibility in controlling dose effects. The risk for overdosing may be higher. In cases of increased liver function the metabolisation rate and the level of active metabolites are also increased (Kreek, 1996). LAAM should be considered for patients only who are already well stabilised on oral Methadone. The recommended doses are 1.2–1.3 times higher than the Methadone doses (Kreek, 1996). Switching from Methadone to LAAM can eventually lead temporarily to withdrawal symptoms, due to the retarded action.

Following 10 cases of life-threatening cases of cardiac disorders in patients treated with LAAM (brand name Orlaam), the European Medicines Evaluation Agency EMEA decided to advise prescribers not to introduce new patients to this therapy. Orlaam has a potential to increase the QTc interval and to be proarrhythmic (EMEA, 2001).

Morphine

Morphine has no important place in substitution treatment. The oral slow-release preparation MST Continus (morphini sulfas pentahydricus) is used as an alternative to oral Methadone in cases where it has unpleasant side-effects. The recommended dose is 600–900 mg per day (Seidenberg and Honegger, 1998).

When intravenously applied, morphine provokes histamine-like local or generalised side-effects. The Amsterdam pilot project prescribing intravenous morphine to a group of highly problematic heroin addicts was discontinued, in part on the basis of such side-effects (van Brussel, 1995). The Swiss project on medical prescription of narcotics also included intravenous morphine which proved to be poorly accepted, due to frequent and partially serious side-effects (Uchtenhagen et al., 1999).

Codeine

5–20% of Codeine is metabolised into morphine. Around 10% in the general population do not have the Iso-enzyme needed for this process (Cytochrome P-450 2D6). In these persons Codeine has not the intended pharmacological effect.

The action of Codeine is better controllable in comparison to Methadone, Codeine having a shorter half-life. Also it has less dependence producing potential. It can be reduced and stopped with less problems. A disadvantage is its irritating effects on the stomach. The indication is mainly limited to patients who need low dosages of substitution drugs.

Clinical experience with Codeine was especially made in Germany when substitution with Methadone was discouraged and restricted. Therapeutic results have been described to be equivalent to those in Methadone substitution treatment (Verthein et al., 1996).

Buprenorphine

Buprenorphine is a synthetic drug derived from Thebaine. It has mixed agonist-antagonist properties. With increased doses the opioid-like effects are reduced, probably due to the increased antagonist effects. When applied sublingually the maximum plasma levels are reached after 2–4 hours. Half-life values for elimination are 3–5 hours. Duration of action increases with dosage. Respiratory depression is minimal. The mortality risk is comparatively low (Walsh et al., 1994). Bioavailability is much lower when applied orally as compared to sublingual application. Dose reduction and termination of treatment is followed by comparatively few withdrawal symptoms (Mattick et al., 1998).

These findings have led to an increased interest for Buprenorphine as an alternative to oral Methadone. It is the substitution drug of choice in France where every physician is entitled to prescribe it. The most frequently used dose is 8 mg per day. The highest dose having no increased risk is mentioned to be 32 mg per day (Mattick et al., 1998). Prescribing the double dose every second day seems feasible without negative consequences. This is seen as one of the advantages (Chadderton, 2000).

Therapeutic outcome is considered to be equivalent in comparison to oral Methadone treatment, measured by retention rates and by a reduction of illegal substance use. There are doubts however with respect to patients who need higher doses of substitution drugs (Mattick et al., 1998). Randomised trials resulted in divergent findings. These may partially be explained by the use of rigid dose schemes and insufficient doses (overview by Mattick et al., 1998). The induction to Buprenorphine takes longer and has more drop-outs in comparison to methadone (Chadderton, 2000).

At intake, direct observation requires several minutes in order to ensure the dissolution of the sub-lingual preparation and thus to prevent intravenous injection after leaving the doctor's office or the clinic (Chadderton, 2000).

Such misuse of Buprenorphine was in fact reported from New Zealand, Australia and Scotland. It has been attempted to prevent such misuse by prescribing a combination of Buprenorphine and Naloxon (Robinson et al., 1993). Double-blind randomised controlled studies have compared daily with intermittent (3 times weekly) administration of Naltrexone (2 mg) in addition to Buprenorphine (8 mg). Intermittent administration of Naltrexone was preferred over daily administration by patients, but a triple crossover trial could not detect differences in drug use, and 45% of urine tests were positive for opiates (Amass et al., 2000, 2001). Buprenorphine plus Naloxone (in a 4:1 combination injected intravenously) was found to produce antagonist-like effects, which was considered to have a potential to reduce intravenous use of Buprenorphine (Fudala et al., 1998). This finding was confirmed in another study using combinations of Buprenorphine and Naloxone (2:1 and 4:1) by intravenous route, registering unpleasant antagonist-like effects and elevated withdrawal symptoms (Mendelson et al., 1999). The present state of knowledge asserts that adding Naloxone to Buprenorphine will precipitate withdrawal when injected in a moderately to severely dependent person, while Naloxone is absorbed sublingually only by 10% and therefore will not block the Buprenorphine effects when applied by the sublingual route (Elkashef, 2002).

Diacetylmorphine (Heroin)

Diacetylmorphine is a highly effective analgesic with a short duration of 4–5 hours and an elimination half-life of a half hour. Monoacetylmorphine and morphine are the active metabolites. If applied intravenously the plasma half-life is 20–30 minutes and the duration of effect 3–4 hours. It passes easily the blood-brain barrier.

A substitution of street heroin by pharmaceutical heroin is practiced in England since decades. Special clinics were set up in the late sixties in urban areas, especially in London. The heroin was handed out by pharmacies on the basis of prescriptions issued by the clinics. Since the early seventies this practice was continously reduced, in favour of prescribing oral and, less frequently, also injectable Methadone (Strang and Gossop, 1996).

In a national Swiss cohort study injectable heroin is prescribed to chronic patients who failed in other previous treatments. The individual doses are on average 471 mg per day, administered in 2–4 intravenous injections under visual control in the clinics. Injectable heroin is often combined with oral Methadone in order to reduce the number of injections per day. This facilitates vocational and social integration of patients, as their day program is not interrupted. Side-effects are histamine-like reactions as is the case with morphine. In some cases cerebral seizures are observed following the injection, in patients with or without previous epilepsy. Patients who are unable to inject because their veins are opliterated or inflamed received in a pilot phase heroin impregnated tobacco-free cigarettes. Because of their low bio-availability of 10% only, these cigarettes were replaced by slow-release heroin tablets (Uchtenhagen et al., 1999).

The Netherlands conducted a randomised trial of prescribing oral Methadone with and without injectable or inhalable heroin for a predefined period of time (van Brussel, 1995; van den Brink et al., 2002).

Indication criteria for the choice of substitution drugs

The present state of evidence does not allow for a formulation of well founded indication criteria. Oral Methadone still is the standard, and other substances are mainly used if Methadone for one reason or another cannot be used or proved to be unsatisfactory. The only exception so far is Buprenorphine which by some is preferred for a substitution treatment of persons who need rather low doses, for adolescents and young adults, and for non injecting heroin dependent persons.

Outcome of substitution treatment

Most outcome studies concern heroin substitution by oral Methadone. Overviews on research results have been presented by the National Institute of Drug Abuse NIDA in the USA (Cooper et al., 1983), by the World Health Organisation (Senay and Uchtenhagen, 1990) and in an Australian reference book (Ward et al., 1998). Although hundreds of outcome studies have been published, the need for more rigorous evaluation still persists.

Effects of *long-term substitution treatment* using oral Methadone were examined in a large number of studies. The early randomised trials and later clinical studies (overview by Ward et al., 1998) have evidenced the following positive results: reduction of illegal drug use, reduction of needle/syringe sharing, reduction in morbidity (especially in blood-born infections) and mortality, improvements in health status, reduction of contacts with drug users, reduction of drug-related delinquency, reintegration into the labour market and an overall normalisation of life-styles. These positive effects have been confirmed by the World Health Organisation (WHO, 1998).

The "classical" evaluation studies using a control group design have documented significant reductions in daily heroin consumption and in arrest rates. Naturalistic studies without control groups often give inferior results; this is explained by the more selective procedures for participants and by a better treatment and care quality in the randomised studies. Also, in the earlier years the rules for running Methadone programmes were more strict and strictly applied.

Comparative cohort studies without a control group design on Methadone substitution treatment, drug-free out-patient treatment and residential treatment have been implemented on a large scale especially in the USA: Drug Abuse Reporting Program DARP (Simpson and Sells, 1990), Treatment Outcome Prospective Study TOPS (Hubbard et al., 1989) and Drug Abuse

Treatment Outcome Study DATOS (Simpson and Curry, 1997). Similar national cohort studies were made in Switzerland (Uchtenhagen and Zimmer-Höfler, 1985) and recently in England (National Treatment Outcome Research Study NTORS, Gossop, 1998). The main findings of these studies are: methadone substitution treatment attracts and serves many more patients than drug-free treatments, and they suffer less from premature dropping-out of patients. There are no consistent findings on differences in therapeutic effects as measured by a reduction in heroin use and in drug-related delinquency. Residential drug-free long-term treatment (mostly in Therapeutic Communities) have best results in achieving a socially integrated drug-free life-style. The least favourable results are documented from out-patient drug-free treatment.

Recent research focused on comparisons of various types of Methadone programmes, intending an identification of predictors for outcome and aiming at an improvement of the programmes. Comparative analysis has identified insufficient Methadone doses as a major reason for therapeutic failure and especially for continued heroin use. Retention and reduction in heroin use could be predicted on the basis of dosage policy. Other relevant factors are the availability of ancillary care services (Ball and Ross, 1991; McLellan et al., 1993) and a flexible duration of treatment. Bureaucratic limitation of treatment duration proved to be counterproductive in terms of relapse rates (Caplehorn, 1994). It is worth mentioning that improvements may occur still after years in substitution treatment. Factors which impair the prognosis are polydrug dependence, personality disorders and non drug-related early delinquency.

New research also concerns the prescription of pharmaceutical heroin as a substitution for street heroin. The British practice has been rarely researched. The one randomised study found lower drop-out rates in the group on injectable heroin, but no clear difference in therapeutic results, as compared to oral Methadone (Hartnoll et al., 1985). A recent study documents the feasibility of prescribing injectable heroin and Methadone (Metrebian et al., 1998). An overview of all programs which prescribed injectable heroin or morphine was presented in 1990 (Mino, 1990).

A national Swiss cohort study was started in 1994 comparing groups receiving injectable morphine, Methadone or heroin, in the framework of a comprehensive assessment and care programme. Entry criteria included multiple failed previous treatment attempts in drug-free programmes or Methadone substitution. Short randomised periods were used in order to identify differences in pharmacological effects and side-effects. The overall cohort was compared to a cohort of new entries into oral Methadone programmes, using the same research protocol. A total of 1,035 patients were enrolled in the cohort receiving injectables, with an average age of 30.8 and an average duration of heroin use of 10.5 years.

The main results of the study were (Uchtenhagen et al., 1999):

— In the randomised substudies the heroin group was found to have better acceptability (recruitment rates), retention rates and reduction of illegal drug use

- Injectable heroin allows for stable dosages as well as oral medication
- In the total cohort there was a rapid improvement in health status, a reduction in illegal and non-prescribed substance use, in contacts with drug users and in drug-related delinquency
- There was no fatal overdose from prescribed substances
- Illegal heroin- and cocaine use showed significant more reduction in comparison to the oral Methadone cohort
- Heroin prescription programmes received good acceptance with authorities and in the general population as evidenced in repeated local and national referenda.

The research protocol, its implementation and the results were examined by an international expert committee, which was nominated by World Health Organisation. The positive results for patients and the feasibility and safety of the programmes were confirmed, however the specific role of heroin prescription could not be identified by lack of a consistent randomisation design. The Committee made recommendations for further research in the field (Ali et al., 1998).

Based on the Swiss study, on a randomised trial in the Netherlands (van Ree, 1998) and the plans for another randomised trial in Germany, the international debate on prescribing pharmaceutical heroin has intensified. Among those engaging in such projects, the main objective is to supplement the already available treatment modalities by an additional one for those who failed in other treatments, while oral Methadone is still perceived to be the drug of choice for substitution purposes. The scientific debate focuses on the place of heroin prescription within the range of treatment options (Bammer et al., 1999).

The Dutch trials on medical co-prescription of heroin to patients in Methadone maintenance treatment (trial duration of 12 months, application of injectable resp. Inhalable heroin) came to the following conclusions:

- The study was conducted and analysed successfully
- Supervised co-prescription of heroin to chronic, treatment-resistant heroin dependent and methadone treated patients is more effective than the continuation of methadone alone
- Supervised co-prescription of heroin to chronic, treatment-resistant heroin dependent and methadone treated patients yields clinically relevant health benefits (physical health and mental status as well as in the social domains)
- The beneficial effects of supervised co-prescription of heroin are linked to the continuation of treatment (81–87% of treatment responders deteriorated substantially following the discontinuation of heroin prescription)
- Supervised co-prescription of heroin is practicable with no excess of serious medical adverse events and with a limited number of controllable public order problems
- The costs of the medical prescription of heroin are dependent on the type of treatment implementation (€ 15,000–20,000 per treatment year per patient).

On the basis of these findings, it was recommended to register heroin as a pharmaceutical product, to introduce supervised co-prescription of heroin to chronic, treatment-resistant heroin dependent and methadone treated patients as a last-resort pharmacotherapeutic option under stringent conditions, to develop a quality assurance system and to implement a follow-up study (van den Brink et al., 2002).

Substitution treatment in an international perspective

A first overview on policy and practice in Methadone substitution treatment in an international perspective was prepared by World Health Organisation (Arif and Westermeyer, 1990). A more recent overview on the legislation, regulations and practice of Methadone substitution in 12 Member States of the European Union was mandated by the European Commission (EMCDDA, 2000). The latter contains detailed descriptions on the basis of information provided by key informants.

Europe has seen a major increase of Methadone substitution treatment and of the respective treatment programmes, as a consequence of the HIV epidemic and especially as a consequence of an increased prevalence of AIDS cases among drug injectors and among their sexual partners. The estimated number of addicts in methadone-substitution treatment has increased 1993–1997 substantially in the European Union: from ca. 400 to ca. 2100 per 100,000 population age 16–60. The largest increase is seen in Spain, Ireland, Italy and — starting from lower figures — Belgium and Germany.

The number of treatment slots is highest, in proportion to the total population, in Spain, Ireland and the Netherlands, followed by Italy, Belgium and the UK. Between 10 and over 200 slots per 100,000 inhabitants (age 16 to 60) are available. There are differences regarding regional distribution and waiting lists.

Another world wide survey was made on behalf of Health Canada (Ruel, 1996), including information from 24 countries. In relation to population figures, Methadone substitution was found to be most frequently available in Switzerland and Hong Kong, followed by Australia, Belgium and the Netherlands.

The international debate on substitution treatment has changed over time. Strict refusal to prescribe substitution drugs on the basis of rather ideological arguments has become quite rare, and the awareness for the needs of a secure and effective implementation has increased. A first attempt was made by World Health Organisation by producing an expert report on the options for the use of substitution treatment in detoxification and maintenance, listing advantages and disadvantages (WHO, 1989). According to this report, the most important advantages were the high potential to recruit dependents into treatment, the comparatively low drop-out rates and the low selectivity, while (avoidable) disadvantages were a diversion of prescribed drugs into the illegal market, endless duration of treatment and the respective costs.

The specific risks of prescribing a narcotic substance for substitution of heroin were already mentioned in the first treatment protocol (Dole and Nyswander, 1965). They considered especially respiratory depression from overdose and deviation into the illegal market. The respective regulations were respected in the first Methadone programmes: visually controlled intake of Methadone, adequate medical and psychosocial care, urine controls for non-prescribed substances. These regulations were reduced or completely abandoned, for economic reasons or in order to lower the threshold for patients. Especially after the arrival of the HIV epidemic so-called low-threshold Methadone substitution was introduced in some places. At present, the modalities how substitution is practised differ in so many respects that the report from the European Commission could state, as the most significant finding, a lack of binding treatment protocols, regulations, monitoring systems and evaluation guidelines (Farrell et al., 1996). An overview of regulations in force by end of 1995 is provided in Table 1 (based on information from Ruel et al., 1996).

The most frequently applied rules are: limitations for handing out Methadone on a take-out basis and controlling non prescribed substance use by urine analysis. Less frequent are dose restrictions, special authorisation needed for prescribing, and a central registration of persons receiving Methadone. Only a minority of countries knows detailed national treatment standards or at least recommendations for good substitution practice. Such provisions have been made for example in Switzerland (Federal Office of Health, 1985, 1995), USA (Parrino, 1991; NIH, 1998) and Germany (Bühringer et al., 1995).

The place of substitution treatment in a therapeutic network

The old debate if substitution treatment is acceptable or not is replaced by a debate on how substitution treatment can be implemented in a helpful way among other treatment approaches for heroin dependent persons.

Originally conceived as a treatment of second choice (in cases where drug-free treatment failed), substitution treatment is nowadays one of the main pillars in the management of heroin dependence. Many more patients prefer substitution treatment over residential drug-free treatment, especially those who still have jobs and a satisfactory social network. Other groups are those who feel discriminated or exposed in the context of residential programmes (e.g. young females, dual diagnosis patients, patients from ethnic minorities with language problems) and also patients who have tried drug-free treatment without positive results. Such obstacles to utilisation can be observed also where access to substitution is appropriate. Wherever heroin dependence is a problem for Public Health and Public Order, substitution treatment therefore is one of the most effective measures not only to improve the situation of the patients, but also to reduce the public problems.

Substitution treatment does not necessarily lead to reduced applications for drug-free treatment. The more patients are substituted, the more will need

Table 1. Regulations for methadone substitution treatment (after Ruel et al., 1996)

	Australia	Canada	Denmark	England	Finland	France	Germany	Hong Kong	Hungary	Israel	Italy	Mexico	Netherlands	New Zealand	Spain	Sweden	Switzerland	USA
Central registration of patients	✗	✗	✗	✗			✗	✗					✗			✗	✗	
Urine controls mandatory	✗	✗	✗	✗	✗	✗	✗	✗		✗	✗	✗	✗	✗	✗	✗	✗	✗
Maximum dose per day		✗	✗	✗		✗	✗			✗		✗	✗	✗	✗		✗	✗
Restricted take-out policy	✗	✗	✗	✗	✗		✗	✗		✗	✗	✗	✗	✗	✗	✗	✗	✗
Special authorisation required	✗	✗			✗		✗		✗	✗		✗		✗	✗	✗	✗	✗
Maximum patient load per prescribing physician	✗	✗					✗			✗	✗	✗		✗				
Maximum patient load per clinic	✗									✗				✗		✗		
Authorisation for specialised clinics only					✗				✗	✗		✗			✗	✗		✗
Authorisation only for physicians specialising in addiction treatment					✗				✗	✗		✗			✗	✗		

detoxification treatment in the end, and the more will look out for drug-free treatment if they are not satisfied with substitution. On the other hand, many who were unsuccessfully in drug-free treatment can be well cared for in substitution treatment. In addition to a meaningful co-existence of therapeutic approaches there are also programmes which offer a mix of approaches: Therapeutic Communities accepting Methadone patients, and Methadone programmes using methods developed in Therapeutic Communities especially for day programmes or semi-residential programmes.

A well functioning integration of approaches and services in a regional network is feasible if there is a political will to support this tendency in order to reach a maximum proportion of dependent persons, and an educational effort for staff concerned in order to improve knowledge on the potential of all therapeutic options and to improve co-ordination and collaboration.

Unsolved problems

One of the most frequent problems arising in substitution treatment is the simultaneous use of non-prescribed substances (Best et al., 2000; Westermann et al., 2000). In the forefront are Benzodiazepines, cocaine and alcohol. Polydrug use increases the mortality risk considerably. It also undermines the efforts to reorient the lifestyle of patients. New ways how to deal with polydrug use must be developed and tested.

Another problem are the high relapse rates which are sometimes found after termination of substitution treatment. Relapse is more frequent after a short duration of treatment, or if duration follows administrative reasons rather than the individual needs of patients. A majority of patients needs adequate psychosocial and rehabilitative measures in order to prevent relapse, which is often in conflict with the need to keep down treatment costs.

A majority of treatment failure seems to be due to insufficient treatment quality. This includes inadequate diagnostic assessment when starting treatment, deficits in psychosocial care and deficient dosage. Many programmes would need improved conditions and increased resources for coping with these demands, but at the same time they suffer from cutting down budgets. A major improvement would be the implementation of binding treatment standards, as is the case in other medical fields.

Ambivalence in attitudes towards substitution treatment however has other roots as well. There is no motivation to substitute a drug of abuse if use and abuse are mainly considered to be irresponsible behaviour that must be punished or at least not gratified. And also there is little motivation if the subjective expectations of users for positive effects of their use are ignored. An evidence based policy looking out for pragmatic approaches and proper evaluation of such approaches is needed in order to overcome the problems outlined here.

References

Arif A, Westermeyer J (1990) Methadone maintenance in the management of opioid dependence. An international review. Praeger, New York

Ali R, Auriacombe M, Casas M, Cottler L, Farrell M, Kleiber D, Kreuzer A, Ogborne A, Rehm J, Ward P (1998) Report of the external panel on the evaluation of the Swiss scientific studies of medically prescribed narcotics to drug addicts. Report to World Health Organisation, Geneva

Amass L, Kamien JB, Mikulich SK (2000) Efficacy of daily and alternate-day dosing regimens with the combination buprenorphine-naloxone tablet. Drug Alcohol Depend 58: 143–152

Amass L, Kamien JB, Mikulich SK (2001) Thrice-weekly supervised dosing with the combination buprenorphine-naloxone tablet is preferred to daily supervised dosing by opiate-dependent humans. Drug Alcohol Depend 61: 173–181

Ball JC, Ross A (1991) The effectiveness of methadone maintenance treatment. Springer, New York

Bammer G, Dobler-Mikola A, Fleming PH, Strang J, Uchtenhagen A (1999) The heroin prescribing debate: integrating science and politics. Science 284: 1277–1278

Bertschy G (1995) Pratique des traitements à la méthadone, Masson, Paris

Best D, Harris J, Gossop M, Farrell M, Finch E, Noble A, Strang J (2000) Use of non-prescribed methadone and other illicit drugs during methadone maintenance treatment. Drug Alcohol Rev 19: 9–16

Brussel G van (1995) Le programme de distribution de morphine a Amsterdam: experiences pratiques. In: Rihs-Middel M, Clerc J, Stamm R (eds) La préscription de stupéfiants sous contrôle médical. Editions Médecine et Hygiène, Genève, pp 161–167

Bühringer G, Gastpar M, Heinz W, Kovar KA, Ladewig D, Naber D, Täschner KL, Uchtenhagen A, Wanke K (1995) Methadon-Standards. Vorschläge zur Qualitätssicherung bei der Methadonsubstitutionim Rahmen der Behandlung von Drogenabhängigen. Enke, Stuttgart

Calsyn DS, Wells EA, Saxon AJ, Jackson TR, Wrede AF, Stanton V, Fleming C (1994) Contingency management of urinalysis results and intensity of counseling services have an interactive impact on methadone maintenance treatment outcome. J Addict Dis 13: 47–63

Caplehorn JR (1994) A comparison of abstinence-oriented and indefinite methadone maintenance treatment. Int J Addict 29: 1361–1375

Chadderton A (2000) Clinical issues in using buprenorphine in the treatment of opiate dependence. Drug Alc Rev 19: 329–335

Chutuape MA, Silverman K, Stitzer ML (1998) Survey assessment of methadone treatment services as reinforcers. Am J Drug Alcohol Abuse 24: 1–16

Cooper JR, Altman F, Brown BS, Czechowicz D (1983) Research on the treatment of narcotic addiction. The state of the art. National Institute on Drug Abuse, Rockville

Dees SM, Dansereau DF, Simpson DD (1997) Mapping-enhanced drug abuse counseling: urinalysis results in the first year of methadone treatment. J Subst Abuse Treat 14: 45–54

Dolan K, Hall W, Wodak A (1998) The provision of methadone within prison settings. In: Ward J, Mattick RP, Hall W (eds) Methadone maintenance treatment and other opioid replacement therapies. Harwood, Amsterdam, pp 379–396

Dole V, Nyswander M (1965) A medical treatment for Diacetylmorphine (heroin) addiction. JAMA 193: 146–150

Elkashef A (2002) Medications for the treatment of opiate dependence in the US. Current therapies and new developments. Communication in WHO Meeting, April 2002

EMCDDA (2000) Reviewing current practice in drug-substitution treatment in the European Union. European Monitoring Centre for Drugs and Drug Addiction EMCDDA, Lisbon

EMEA (2001) Public statement on the recommendation to suspend the marketing authorisation for Orlaam in the European Union. European Agency for the Evaluation of Medicinal Products, London

Finnegan LP, Hagan T, Kaltenbach KA (1991) Scientific foundation of clinical practice: opiate use in pregnant women. Bull NY Acad Med 67: 223–239

Fudala PJ, Yu E, Macfadden W, Boardman C, Ciang CN (1998) Effects of buprenorphine and naloxone in morphine-stabilised opioid addicts. Drug Alcohol Depend 50: 1–8

Gossop M (1998) NTORS at one year. The National Treatment Outcome Research Study. Department of Health, London

Hartnoll R, Mitcheson M, Battersby A, Brown G, Ellis M, Fleming P, Hedley N (1980) Evaluation of heroin maintenance in a controlled trial. Arch Gen Psychiatry 37: 877–884

Hubbard RL, Marsden ME, Rachal JV, Haarwood HJ, Cavanaugh ER, Ginzburg HM (1989) Drug abuse treatment. A national study of effectiveness. University of North Carolina Press, Chapel Hill

Kreek MJ (1996) Long-term pharmacotherapy for opiate (primarily heroin) addiction: opioid agonists. In: Schuster CH, Kuhar MJ (eds) Pharmacological aspects of drug dependence. Toward an integrated neurobehavioral approach. Springer, Berlin Heidelberg New York Tokyo, pp 487–562

Lifschitz MH, Wilson GS, Smith EO, Desmond MM (1985) Factors affecting head growth and intellectual function in children of drug addicts. Pediatrics 75: 269–274

Ling W, Klett JC, Gillis RC (1980) A cooperative clinical study of methadyl acetate. Arch Gen Psychiatry 37: 908–911

McLellan AT, Arndt IO, Metzger IS, Woody GE, O'Brien CP (1993) The effects of psychosocial services in substance abuse treatment. JAMA 269: 1953–1959

Maddux JF, Desmond DP, Esquivel M (1995) Rapid admission and retention on methadone. Am J Drug Alcohol Abuse 21: 533–547

Mattick RP, Oliphant D, Ward J, Hall W (1998) The effectiveness of other opioid replacement therapies: LAAM, Heroin, Buprenorphine, Naltrexone and injectable maintenance. In: Ward J, Mattick RP, Hall W (eds) Methadone maintenance treatment and other opioid replacement therapies. Harwood, Amsterdam, pp 123–160

Mendelson J, Jones RT, Welm S, Baggott M, Fernandez I, Melby AK, Nath RP (1999) Buprenorphine and naloxone combinations: the effects of three dose ratios in morphine-stabilised, opiate dependent volunteers. Psychopharmacology 141: 37–46

Metrebian N, Shanahan W, Wells B, Stimson GV (1998) Feasibility of prescribing injectable heroin and methadone to opiate-dependent drug users: associated health gains and harm reductions. Med J Aust 168: 596–600

Mino A (1990) Analyse scientifique de la littérature sur la remise contrôlée d'héroïne ou de morphine. Institutions universitaires de psychiatrie, Genève

National Institute of Drug Abuse NIDA (1999) Principles of drug addiction treatment. A research-based guide. National Institute of Drug Abuse, National Institutes of Health, Bethesda, MD

National Institutes of Health NIH (1998) National consensus development panel on effective medical treatment of opiate addiction. JAMA 280: 1936–1943

Parrino MW (1991) State Methadone Treatment Guidelines. U.S. Department of Health and Human Services, Rockville

Raschke P (1994) Substitutionstherapie. Ergebnisse langfristiger Behandlung von Opiatabhängigen. Lambertus, Freiburg im Breisgau

Rhee JM van (1998) Study on the effectiveness of medically coprescribed heroin. Progress report. Central Committee on the Treatment of Heroin Addicts, Utrecht

Rhoades HM, Creson D, Elk R, Schmitz J, Grabowsk J (1998) Retention, HIV risk, and illicit drug use during treatment: methadone dose and visit frequency. Am J Publ Health 88: 34–39

Robinson GM, Dukes PD, Robinson BJ, Cook RR, Mahoney GN (1993) The misuse of buprenorphine and buprenorphine-naloxone combination in Wellington, New Zealand. Drug Alcohol Depend 33: 81–86

Ruel JM (1996) International survey on the use of methadone in the treatment of narcotic addiction. Bureau of Drug Surveillance, Ottawa, Canada

Savage C, Karp EG, Curran SF, Hanlon TE, McCabe OL (1976) Methadone/LAAM maintenance: a comparison study. Compr Psychiatry 17: 415–424

Scott RTA, Jay MJH, Keith R, Oliver JS, Cassidy MT (1999) A confidential enquiry into methadone-related deaths. Addiction 94: 1789–1794

Seidenberg A, Honegger U (1998) Methadon, Heroin und andere Opioide. Medizinisches Manual für die ambulante opioidgestützte Behandlung. Huber, Bern

Senay EC, Uchtenhagen A (1990) Methadone in the treatment of opioid dependence. In: Arif A, Westermeyer J (eds) Methadone maintenance in the management of opioid dependence. Praeger, New York, pp 19–54

Senay EC, Barthwell A, Marks R, Bokos PJ (1994) Medical maintenance: an interim report. J Addict Dis 13: 65–69

Simpson DD, Sells SB (1990) Opioid addiction and treatment: a 12-year follow-up. Krieger, Malabar

Simpson DD, Curry SJ (eds) (1997) Drug Abuse Treatment Outcome Study DATOS. Psychol Addict Behav 11 (special issue)

Simpson DD, Joe GW, Dansereau DF, Chatham LR (1997) Strategies for improving methadone treatment process and outcomes. J Drug Issues 27: 239–260

Stitzer ML, Iguchi MY, Felch LJ (1992) Contingent take-home incentive: effects on drug use of methadone. J Consult Clin Psychol 60: 927–934

Strang J, Gossop M (1996) Heroin prescribing in the British system: a historical review. Eur Addict Res 2: 185–193

Svikis DS, Lee JH, Haug NA, Stitzer ML (1997) Attendance incentives for outpatient treatment: effects in methadone- and nonmethadone-maintained pregnant drug dependent women. Drug Alcohol Depend 48: 33–41

Tennant FS, Rawson RA, Pumphrey E, Seecof R (1986) Clinical experiences with 959 opioid-dependent patients treated with levo-alpha-acetylmethadol (LAAM). J Subst Abuse Treatment 3: 195–202

Uchtenhagen A, Zimmer-Höfler D (1985) Heroinabhängige und ihre normalen Altersgenossen. Herkunft, Lebenssituation, Zweijahresverlauf im Quervergleich. Haupt, Bern

Uchtenhagen A, Dobler-Mikola A, Steffen T, Gutzwiller F, Blättler R, Pfeifer S (1999) Prescription of narcotics for heroin addicts. Main results of the Swiss National Cohort Study. Karger, Basel

Van den Brink W, Hendriks VM, Blanken P, Huijsman JA, van Ree JM (2002) Medical co-prescription of heroin. Two randomised controlled trials. Central Committee on the Treatment of Heroin Addicts, Utrecht

Verthein U, Degkwitz P, Haasen C, Raschke P, Krausz M (1996) Die Substitutionsbehandlung Opiatabhängiger mit Codein/Dihydrocodein und Methadon — ein Kontrollgruppenvergleich. Sucht 42: 108–115

Walsh SL, Preston KL, Stitzer ML, Cone EJ, Bigelow GE (1994) Clinical pharmacology of buprenorphine. Ceiling effects at high doses. Clin Pharmacol Ther 55: 569–580

Ward J, Mattick R, Hall W (1998) Methadone maintenance treatment and other opioid replacement therapies. Harwood, Amsterdam

Westermann B, Bellmann G, Jellinek C (eds) (2000) Beigebrauch: offene Grenzen der Substitution. Beltz, Weinheim

Woody GE, McLellan AT, Luborsky LO, Brien CP Psychotherapy in community methadone programs: a validation study. Am J Psychiatry 152: 1302–1308

World Health Organization (1989) Options for the use of methadone in the treatment of drug dependence. Geneva (WHO/MNH/DAT/89/2)
World Health Organisation (1998) WHO Expert Committee on Drug Dependence. Thirtieth Report. WHO, Geneva (Technical Report Series 873)

Author's address: Prof. Dr. A. Uchtenhagen, Addiction Research Institute, Konradstrasse 32, CH-8005 Zurich, Switzerland, e-mail: uchtenhagen@isf.unizh.ch

Designer drugs: how dangerous are they?

L. Reneman

Department of Radiology, Academic Medical Center, Amsterdam, The Netherlands

Summary. Of the designer drugs, the amphetamine analogues are the most popular and extensively studied, ecstasy (3,4-methylenedioxymethamphetamine; MDMA) in particular. They are used recreationally with increasing popularity despite animal studies showing neurotoxic effects to serotonin (5-HT) and/or dopamine (DA) neurones. However, few detailed assessments of risks of these drugs exist in humans. Previously, there were no methods available for directly evaluating the neurotoxic effects of amphetamine analogues in the living human brain. However, development of *in vivo* neuroimaging tools have begun to provide insights into the effects of MDMA in human brain. In this review, contributions of brain imaging studies on the potential 5-HT and/or DA neurotoxic effects of amphetamine analogues will be highlighted in order to delineate the risks these drugs engender in humans, focusing on MDMA. An overview will be given of PET, SPECT and MR Spectroscopy studies employed in human users of these drugs. Most of these studies provide suggestive evidence that MDMA is neurotoxic to 5-HT neurones, and (meth)amphetamine to DA neurones in humans. These effects seem to be dose-related, leading to functional impairments such as memory loss, and are reversible in several brain regions. However most studies have had a retrospective design, in which evidence is indirect and differs in the degree to which any causative links can be implied between drug use and neurotoxicity. Therefore, at this moment, it cannot be ascertained that humans are susceptible to MDMA-induced 5-HT injury or (meth)amphetamine-induced DA injury. Finally, although little is known about other amphetamine analogues there are important questions as to the safety of these designer drugs as well, in view of the fact that they are chemically closely related to MDMA and some have been shown to be 5-HT neurotoxins in animals.

Introduction

There is debate over the initial meaning of the term ‘designer drug’. Some point out that it originally referred to drugs which were made for specific selected effects. However others claim that it is used to describe the private manufacture of synthetic analogues slightly different from parent compounds that, by design, rendered them temporarily immune from the control of the Drug Enforcement Agency (DEA). In the past, changes to a chemical structure would allow a newly synthesized drug to escape regulation until the legal authorities discovered its existence. Since in 1986 the US Government (followed in 1997 by the EU) amended the Controlled Substances Act (CSA) with the "designer drug" legislation, today the DEA can take immediate action and schedule related substances.

Synthetic drugs with long histories of illicit use include amphetamines and lysergic acid diethylamide (LSD), while ecstasy (3,4-methylenedioxymethamphetamine; MDMA) and other drugs listed in Shulgin's Pihkal list (1991) have much shorter histories of illicit use. In the mid 1980's the term designer drug began to be used synonymously with dance or recreational drugs following the emergence of MDMA and other ring-substituted amphetamines in the recreational drug scene, although non-designer drugs such as cannabis and cocaine are also consumed in these settings. This is perhaps why the term designer drug nowadays lacks precision. As popularised by the lay press, the term is often used when referring to 'club drugs'. Club drugs are drugs that have become popular among teens and young adults at dance clubs and "raves", and not only include amphetamine analogues but non-designer drugs as well, such as flunitrazepam (Rohypnol®), gamma-hydroxybutyrate (GHB) and ketamine. However, because of the strong association in the literature with MDMA-like substances, in the present review the term designer drug will be used for synthetic drugs derived from amphetamine and methamphetamine: amphetamine analogues.

Amphetamine analogues are becoming increasing popular among adolescents and young adults. Of these, MDMA is unquestionably the most popular and extensively studied. Its use has shown a dramatic increase over recent years when use of other illicit drugs remained constant or decreased in the US (Strote et al., 2002; Johnston et al., 2002). The greatest concern with respect to the safety of MDMA and related drugs is the large body of animal literature suggesting that these drugs are selective neurotoxins. Studies have shown significant long-lasting neurochemical and morphological changes in serotonin (5-HT) neurones in response to MDMA, changes in dopamine (DA) neurones in response to amphetamine, and changes in both 5-HT and DA neurones in response to methamphetamine treatment. There is also growing concern about the potential manufacture of other and newer designer drugs sold as an alternative of MDMA, or which are added to MDMA tablets.

However, despite the popularity and considerable media attention, few detailed assessments of risks in humans exist. This may be due to the fact that previously, potential neurotoxic changes in the living human brain have only been identified using *indirect* methods. However, *in vivo* neuroimaging tools, such as positron emission tomography (PET), single photon emission computed tomography (SPECT), and several magnetic resonance (MR) imaging applications show great promise in *directly* identifying potential neurotoxic consequences of amphetamine designer drugs in the living human brain.

The goal of this article is to review the available neuroimaging data on potential neurotoxic effects on the 5-HT and DA system of several of the most prevalent amphetamine analogues in order to delineate the risks these drugs engender in humans, focusing on MDMA.

Studying neurotoxicity

The four most widely used biological markers of 5-HT or DA neurotoxicity of amphetamine analogues as indicated by Kieven and Seiden (1989) in animals are:

— Long-lasting depletions in 5-HT or DA levels
— Decrease in 5-HT transporter (SERT) or DA transporter (DAT) densities
— Decreased activity of the synthetic enzymes for 5-HT or DA
— Alterations in neuronal morphology

All these criteria have been studied in animals treated with amphetamine analogues, amphetamine, and methamphetamine. In humans the following biological markers for 5-HT and DA neurotoxicity have been studied using in vivo neuroimaging techniques:

— Decrease in SERT or DAT
— Non-specific neuronal loss: decreases in levels of the neurometabolite *N*-acetylaspartate

Furthermore, if use of amphetamine or its analogues leads to brain pathology, this would result in impairments of functions in which 5-HT or DA play an important role (e.g., cognition, motor speed). Several studies have therefore attempted to investigate:

— An association between biological markers of neuronal damage and behavioural function

Although several neuroimaging studies have investigated whether use of amphetamine analogues and ther parent compound are associated with secondary, indirect, changes in post-synaptic 5-HT and DA receptor densities, brain microvasculature and cerebral glucose metabolic rate, this review will concentrate on the long-term effects of these drugs on the pre-synaptic 5-HT and DA system only.

In vivo neuroimaging techniques

PET and SPECT

The introduction of an increasing number of radioactive tracers and the development of special detecting systems, enable the detection of molecules *in vivo* and the production of functional images of brain chemistry. The most advanced detecting systems nowadays are PET and SPECT. PET uses relatively short-lived positron-emitting isotopes (such as ^{11}C or ^{18}F), whereas SPECT utilises radioligands with a longer half-life (such as ^{123}I and ^{99}mTc).

Spatial resolution of most recently developed PET systems is approximately 4mm. The spatial and temporal resolution of SPECT is lower than that of PET. However, because of the lower costs of the logistics and production of SPECT radiotracers, this technique is more widely available than PET.

SERT and DAT are structural elements of the 5-HT and DA neuron, respectively, and thought to be a reliable marker of the integrity of these neurons (Zhou et al., 1998; Scheffel and Ricaurte 1990; Villemagne et al., 1998). The use of these transporters as an index for neuronal integrity is indicated by findings of decreased brain SERT and DAT levels in animals treated with 5-HT and DA neurotoxins (Battaglia et al., 1987; Scheffel et al., 1998; Koda and Gibb, 1973; Seiden et al., 1976; Bakhit et al., 1981; Ricaurte et al., 1980).

Recently, PET and SPECT radioligands have been developed for neuroimaging of SERT and DAT in the human brain. Because animal studies already showed that MDMA-, and methamphetamine induced neurotoxicity is associated with loss of SERT, while amphetamine and methamphetamine-induced neurotoxicity is associated with loss of DAT, PET and SPECT are ideally suited for studying the potential neurotoxic effects of amphetamine analogues in the living human brain. However, because there are important features for a good *in vivo* tracer for these transporters, there are only a few radioligands (particularly with respect to the SERT) which fulfil at least some of the criteria and subsequently only several tracers have been used to investigate the effects of amphetamine designer drugs *in vivo.*

^{1}H MR Spectroscopy

Another way to investigate potential neurotoxic effects of amphetamine designer drugs, is by studying certain aspects of cerebral biochemistry using proton magnetic resonance spectroscopy (^{1}H MRS). Peaks of *N*-acetyl (NA) groups (primarily *N*-acetylaspartate, NAA), choline-containing compounds (Cho) and creatine plus phosphocreatine (Cr) can be obtained non-invasively. Determination of the myoinositol (MI) peak is also possible using short echo times. NAA is contained almost exclusively within neuronal cell bodies and axons (Howe et al., 1993), and considered a marker for neuronal loss or dysfunction (Urenjak et al., 1993; Higuchi et al., 1997), whereas MI is considered a possible marker for gliosis, reflecting ongoing repair processes.

Methylenedioxy analogues of amphetamine

Of the amphetamine analogues, the three methylenedioxy analogues of amphetamine, namely MDA (3,4-methylenedioxyamphetamine), its *N*-methyl analogue MDMA and *N*-ethyl analogue MDE (3,4-methylenedioxyethyl-amphetamine) are the best known, and collectively termed methylenedioxy analogues of amphetamine. They differ from amphetamine in that they have a methylenedioxy ($-0-CH_2-0-$) group attached to the aromatic ring (i.e., are "ring-substituted"). MDMA and MDA were typical designer drugs until they were added to Schedule I of the US Controlled Drug Act in 1985, followed by MDE in 1986. MDA, MDMA and MDE have very similar effects in humans, but differ in potency, time of onset and duration of action (Hegadoren et al., 1999). They are typically used recreationally at "raves" because they enhance energy, endurance, sociability and sexual arousal, making them particularly popular among youngster.

Although data on the current prevalence of MDA and MDE are sparse, epidemiological studies have shown a dramatic increase in MDMA use over recent years. The prevalence of past year MDMA use among US college students rose from 2.8% to 4.7% between 1997 and 1999, an increase of 69% (Strote et al., 2002). In a 30 year longitudinal study at a large US college it was observed that weekly use of alcohol has remained stable, whereas most illicit drugs declined after a peak in 1978, except for MDMA which increased over the years (Pope et al., 2001). This study also showed that MDMA is the second most frequently tried illicit drug after marijuana. The Monitoring the Future Study (Johnston et al., 2002) has shown for 12th graders in the US that although last year MDMA use continued to increase (around 9% in 2001), the rate of increase began to fall off since 2001. In line with this, MDMA use has generally stabilised in the EU, although upward trends in MDMA use are still observed in some urban areas (EMCDDA 2001). However, the use of MDMA (and methamphetamine) has shown a huge increase in production and use in many Asian countries, like Hong Kong and Indonesia (Ahmad, 2002).

Animal studies

Almost more than two decades ago the first evidence emerged indicating that methylenedioxy analogues of amphetamine produced selective toxic effects on brain 5-HT neurons (Ricaurte et al., 1985). Of the methylenedioxy analogues, MDMA is by far the best studied. Dose-related reductions in brain markers of 5-HT axons, such as 5-HT and 5-hydroxyindolaceticacid (5-HIAA) (Commins et al., 1987; Schmidt et al., 1987a, 1986; Stone et al., 1986), SERT density (Battaglia et al., 1987; Commins et al., 1987) and the activity of tryptophan hydroxylase (Schmidt et al., 1987b; Stone, 1986) have consistently been reported in animals treated with MDMA. Similar observations have been made for MDA and MDE, even though MDE has been shown to be a less potent neurotoxin (Gibb, 1987; Johnson et al., 1986; Kamien et al., 1986; Stone et al., 1987).

MDMA-induced neurochemical deficits, which last well beyond the period of drug administration, have been correlated with the disappearance of 5-HT immunoreactive axons (Molliver et al., 1990; O'Hearn et al., 1988; Wilson et al., 1989) and have been confirmed using silver impregnation of degenerating neurons (Commins et al., 1987).

Neurotoxic effects of MDMA on 5-HT neurons have been demonstrated in a variety of animal species. The magnitude and duration of MDMA's effects are dependent upon the dose and number of injections given (Steele et al., 1994). Primates are much more vulnerable to the neurotoxic actions of MDMA than rodents. A single dose of 5 mg/kg MDMA has been shown to produce long-lasting depletion of 5-HT in monkey brain (Ricaurte et al., 1988). Brain levels of dopamine and its metabolite are not reduced by low doses of MDMA, but are depleted after higher doses (Commins et al., 1987), suggesting that while MDMA is more toxic to 5-HT than dopaminergic systems, it can also damage dopamine neurons. Interestingly, it has recently been shown that a closely spaced but low-dose regimen leads to severe dopaminergic neurotoxicity in addition to less pronounced serotonergic neurotoxicity in primates (Ricaurte et al., 2002). MDMA neurotoxicity was associated with increased vulnerability to motor dysfunction.

There is evidence indicating that 5-HT rich brain regions differ in their sensitivity to MDMA neurotoxic effects. Areas rich in 5-HT terminals such as the cerebral cortex show more severe deficits than brain regions containing fibers of passage (hypothalamus) or cell bodies (brain stem) (Commins et al., 1987; O'Hearn et al., 1988). Some evidence exists that the 5-HT system of rats is able to recover within six months to one year following repeated injections with 10 or 20 mg/kg MDMA (Battaglia et al., 1988; Scanzello et al., 1993). In non-human primates the neurotoxic effects of MDMA may be permanent in some (particularly cortical) brain regions (Hatzidimitriou et al., 1999; Ricaurte et al., 1992a,b) while other brain regions (hypothalamus and thalamus) show evidence of complete recovery. It has been suggested that the distance of the affected axon terminal field from the rostral raphe nuclei influences recovery of 5-HT axons after MDMA injury (Hatzidimitriou et al., 1999).

These observations in animals seem to be relevant to humans, since doses used by humans fall squarely into the range of dosages that are toxic in animals, when dosages are adjusted to account for interspecies differences (Ricaurte et al., 2000). The observation that smaller animal species require higher doses of drug to achieve equivalent drug effects is predicted by the principle of interspecies scaling. This method utilizes known relations between body mass/surface area and accounts for differences in drug clearance (Mordenti and Chappell, 1989).

Human studies

In humans, of all three methylenedioxy analogues, only the effects of MDMA on 5-HT neurons has been studied. Studies have been conducted in human MDE users, but these concerned brain microvasculature and cerebral glucose metabolic rate, which fall beyond the scope of this overview.

PET

Trans-1,2,3,5,6,10-β-hexahydro-6-[4-(methylthio)phenyl] pyrrolo-[2,1-α]isoquinoline ([^{11}C]McN5652) is the first PET radioligand successfully developed in 1992 to label SERTs in the living human brain (Boja et al., 1992). *In vitro*, the active enantiomer (+)-[^{11}C]McN5652 binds selectively to SERTs, whereas the uptake of the inactive enantiomer (−)-[^{11}C]McN5652 is relatively uniform across brain regions. Scheffel and co-workers (1998) were the first to validate the use of [^{11}C]McN5652 PET in detecting MDMA-induced 5-HT neuronal loss in an MDMA-treated baboon. Mean radioactivity of (+)-[^{11}C]McN5652, but not (−)[^{11}C]McN5652, was reduced in all brain regions studied, ranging from 44% in the pons to 89% in the occipital cortex. Data obtained from PET studies correlated well with regional 5-HT axonal marker concentrations in the CNS measured after sacrifice of the animal, although [^{11}C]McN5652 PET tended to underestimate the extent of 5-HT damage found post-mortem. Therefore, is was concluded that using [^{11}C]McN5652 PET it should be possible to determine whether human MDMA users are susceptible to MDMA's neurotoxic effects.

Subsequently, after having validated [^{11}C]McN5652 PET for detecting MDMA-induced 5-HT neuronal loss, a PET study with [^{11}C]McN5652 was carried out in 1998 in human MDMA users (McCann et al., 1998a). The purpose of the study was to compare [^{11}C]McN5652 labelled SERT densities in human MDMA users with SERT densities in control subjects. Nine males and 4 females who reported previous use of MDMA were enrolled, along with 9 male and 6 female control subjects. Participants agreed to abstain from use of psychoactive drugs for at least 3 weeks before the study. As in the MDMA-treated baboon, global decreases in SERT densities were observed in the MDMA users, which correlated with the extent of previous MDMA use. Taken in conjunction with the results of previous animal studies showing selective decreases in 5-HT axonal markers after treatment with MDMA (Scheffel et al., 1998), this was the first report providing direct evidence that MDMA users are susceptible to MDMA-induced brain 5-HT neuronal injury.

SPECT

Using SPECT both the 5-HT and DA-system have been investigated in MDMA users.

5-HT system Since then, similar observations have been made using [^{123}I]β-CIT SPECT. The cocaine analogue 2β-carbomethoxy-3β-(4-iodophenyl)tropane (β-CIT) is presently the best studied and most used SPECT tracer for labelling of SERTs. [^{11}C]β-CIT binds with high affinity to both DAT and SERTs (Boja et al., 1991). The specific uptake of [^{123}I]β-CIT in the striatum is primarily associated with DAT, since it is blocked by the selective DA uptake inhibitor GBR 12,909 but not by selective 5-HT uptake inhibitors (Laruelle et al., 1993). By contrast, uptake of β-CIT in 5-HT rich brain regions such as the brainstem, thalamus and cerebral cortex can be blocked by 5-HT uptake inhibitors (Farde et al., 1994; Kuikka et al., 1995; Laruelle et al., 1993). Thus, these studies indicate that in selected brain areas (e.g., brainstem, thalamus, and possibly cerebral cortex) in which SERT densities exceed those of DAT, it is possible to estimate SERT densities using [^{123}I]β-CIT.

Ex vivo and *in vitro* studies in animals have shown that [^{123}I]β-CIT adequately detects changes in cortical as well as subcortical SERT densities secondary to 5-HT neurotoxicity (Lew et al., 1996; Scheffel et al., 1992). To validate the use of [^{123}I]β-CIT in combination with SPECT in detecting 5-HT neurotoxic lesions, recently a study was undertaken in a rhesus monkey (Reneman et al., 2002a). Following baseline [^{123}I]β-CIT SPECT scans, the monkey was treated with MDMA. SPECT studies at 4, 10 and 31 days post-MDMA treatment revealed decreases in [^{123}I]β-CIT binding ratios in the hypothalamic/midbrain region. Data obtained from SPECT studies in this brain region correlated well with regional SERT densities obtained with autoradiography after sacrifice of the animal.

Several studies have recently been conducted using [^{123}I]β-CIT SPECT to study the effects of MDMA on human brain 5-HT neurons. Semple and colleagues (1999) observed decreased [^{123}I]β-CIT binding only in the cerebral cortex (particularly prominent in the primary sensory cortex) of 10 male MDMA users as compared to 10 well-matched controls. Reductions in binding inversely correlated with time since last MDMA use. No correlations were observed between [^{123}I]β-CIT binding ratios and a variety of neuropsychological measures. However, there are several problems associated with this study. Subjects were asked to abstain from psychoactive drugs for one week, whereas this was 3 weeks in the [^{11}C]McN5652 PET study (McCann et al., 1998a). Furthermore, [^{123}I]β-CIT SPECT scans were acquired 90 minutes post injection of the radiotracer. However, [^{123}I]β-CIT does not reach near-equilibrium conditions earlier than about four hours post injection (Pirker et al., 2000). At scanning times this early, factors related to radioligand delivery and washout, rather than SERT binding *per se*, play a prevalent role in determining [^{123}I]β-CIT binding.

Using [^{123}I]β-CIT SPECT, Reneman and colleagues (2001a) replicated findings of previous PET and SPECT studies suggesting that heavy use of MDMA is associated with neurotoxic effects on 5-HT neurons in several 5-HT rich brain regions. Three different subgroups of 54 MDMA users (moderate and heavy users, as well as ex-heavy users) and 15 controls were scanned after a drug-free interval of at least 3 weeks. Subjects were recruited from the same community sources, and thus well matched for age, gender distribution and psychosocial factors. Overall tests for group and group by gender were significant, indicating a significant overall effect of MDMA use on [^{123}I]β-CIT binding which was significantly different for males and females. More specifically, [^{123}I]β-CIT binding ratios were significantly decreased in all brain regions studied in female, but not in male, heavy MDMA users, suggesting that females may be more susceptible than males to the neurotoxic effects of MDMA (Fig. 1). In line with this, a significant (negative) association was observed between extent of MDMA exposure with [^{123}I]β-CIT binding in females, but not in males. It was also observed that MDMA-induced neurotoxic changes in most, but not all, brain regions of female ex-MDMA users were reversible, and that moderate MDMA use may lead to neurotoxic changes in the parieto-occipital cortex and occipital cortex, brain regions which seem to be particularly sensitive to MDMA's effects.

Regional differences in SERT densities reported in MDMA users studied with $[^{123}I]\beta$-CIT SPECT by Semple and Reneman are fewer than in the study of McCann and colleagues. This may reflect higher non-specific binding of $[^{123}I]\beta$-CIT. However, data obtained from $[^{123}I]\beta$-CIT SPECT studies in the MDMA treated rhesus monkey correlated well with regional SERT densities obtained with autoradiography in some brain regions (Reneman et al., 2002a). As for $[^{11}C]$McN5652 PET, also $[^{123}I]\beta$-CIT SPECT may lack adequate sensitivity to detect smaller MDMA-induced 5-HT lesions. The presence of SERTs in neocortical regions is well documented in human brain (Backstrom et al., 1989; Gurevich et al., 1996). There has however been some discussion in the literature about the ability of $[^{123}I]\beta$-CIT to bind to SERT in the cerebral cortex, since $[^{123}I]\beta$-CIT lacks selectivity for the SERT. Farde and co-workers (1994) have shown that $[^{11}C]\beta$-CIT uptake in monkey cortex could be displaced by 50% by citalopram, a selective SERT inhibitor, but not by GBR 12909, a selective dopamine transporter inhibitor. These findings are consistent with reports on binding of $[^{123/125}I]\beta$-CIT to SERTs in the neocortex of rats (Boja et al., 1992; Scheffel et al., 1992), suggesting that $[^{123}I]\beta$-CIT very likely binds to SERT in the cerebral cortex. Future studies should be conducted to validate the use of $[^{123}I]\beta$-CIT SPECT in detecting SERT reduction in the cerebral cortex.

DA-system Because tablets sold as "ecstasy" do often not only contain MDMA but other compounds well known to cause dopaminergic neurotoxicity such as (meth)amphetamine, and in view of a recent study suggesting that MDMA can lead to DA neurotoxicity in primates (Ricaurte et al., 2002), it is of interest to study potential DA neurotoxicity in humans.

Using $[^{123}I]\beta$-CIT SPECT, Reneman and colleagues (2002c) compared striatal DAT densities in 29 sole MDMA users and compared them with DAT densities in 15 non-MDMA using control subjects. Subjects were scanned after an abstention period of at least 3 weeks. Striatal DAT densities were significantly increased (+13%) in MDMA users, after adjustment for age. Semple (1999) also did not observe a difference in DAT between 10 MDMA users and 10 controls. These initial observations in humans suggest that sole use of MDMA is not related to dopaminergic neurotoxicity in humans, in contrast to data in primates showing severe DA neurotoxicity in primates exposed to an MDMA regimen modelled after one used by humans (Ricaurte et al., 2002).

^{1}H-MR Spectroscopy

In 1999 Chang and colleagues reported findings on ^{1}H MRS spectra obtained in 22 MDMA users and 37 controls, who had to abstain from psychoactive drugs for at least 2 weeks. Normal NAA levels were observed in MDMA users, but MI and MI/Cr levels were increased in the parietal white matter of MDMA users. The cumulative lifetime MDMA dose showed significant effects of MI in the parietal white matter and the occipital cortex. The normal NAA levels suggest a lack of significant neuronal injury in MDMA users, whereas increased MI may reflect increased glial content, possibly reflecting ongoing repair processes.

In contrast, Reneman and co-workers (2002b) recently reported decreased NAA/Cr and NAA/Cho levels in the frontal cortex of 15 male MDMA users, studied at least 1 week after the last MDMA tablet taken, as compared to 12 gender and age matched control subjects. Furthermore, a significant association was observed between extent of previous MDMA use and NAA/Cr or NAA/Cho ratios in the frontal cortex. Discrepancies between the study by Chang and that of Reneman, may be attributed in part to age-associated differences between both studies. In the Reneman study, subjects (both MDMA users and controls) were on average younger with a smaller age range. However, precise quantification of 'near-water' resonance peaks is difficult in water suppressed ^{1}H MRS, and may therefore also account for the discrepancy between the studies.

Obergriesser and colleagues (2001) compared hippocampal ^{1}H MR Spectroscopic Imaging (MRSI) data of 5 MDMA users with those of 5 controls, after a drug free period of at least 3 weeks. Hippocampal NAA levels and NAA/(Cr + Cho) did not differ between groups.

Linking biological markers of neuronal injury with behavioural function

By combining imaging studies with neuropsychological assessment it is possible to study links between neuronal loss, or brain damage, and cognitive function. If MDMA does produce 5-HT neurotoxicity in humans, there would be important ramifications for the mental health and psychological function of people who use this drug, because irreversible loss of 5-HT neurones may be responsible for an immediate or delayed onset of neuropsychiatric disorders in which 5-HT has been implicated. Specifically, 5-HT imbalance has been postulated to underlie psychiatric disorders including depression, anxiety, panic disorder, and disorders of impulse control. In line with this, there have been many case reports of neuropsychiatric sequelae after MDMA use, including paranoid psychosis, anxiety, depression and panic disorder (Hegadoren et al., 1999; Schifano et al., 1998). Furthermore, since 5-HT appears to play an important role in cognitive function, and greatest neurotoxic effects of MDMA in animals are observed in the frontal cortex and hippocampus — areas known to play crucial roles in cognitive function and memory. Several studies have found an association between markers of neuronal injury and impaired cognitive function in MDMA users. Memory is of particular interest since several studies have found that recreational MDMA users display significant memory impairments, whereas their performance on other cognitive tests is generally normal (Parrott, 2000).

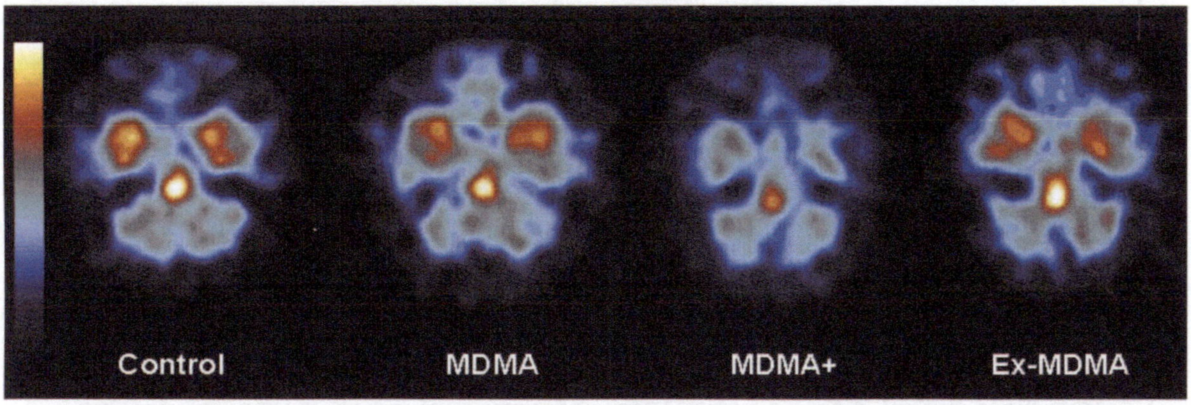

Fig. 1. [^{123}I]β-CIT SPECT images of a female control subject, a female moderate MDMA user (MDMA), a female heavy MDMA user (MDMA+) and a female ex-MDMA user (ex-MDMA). Transverse slices from the brain at the level of the midbrain. In the three images the level of [^{123}I]β-CIT activity is color encoded from low (black) to high (white) and scaled to the maximum in the slice of the control subject. The images show loss of 5-HT transporters in the midbrain of a female heavy MDMA user (from Reneman et al., 2001, with permission)

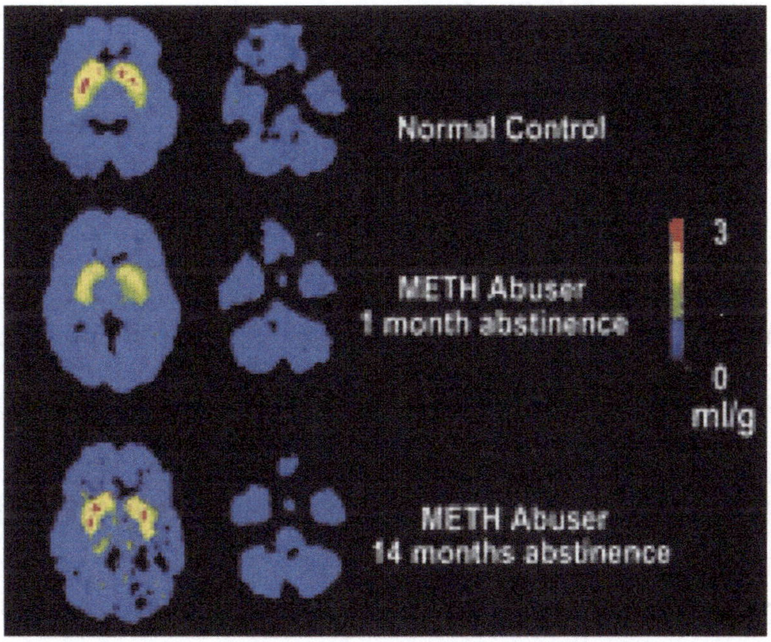

Fig. 2. Brain images of the distribution volume of [^{11}C]*d-threo*-methylphenidate in a control and a methamphetamine abuser. Images shown were obtained at the level of the striatum (images to the *left*) and the cerebellum (images to the *right*), and they are from a normal control and a methamphetamine abuser evaluated twice, during short and protracted abstinence. Notice the significant increases in binding in striatum in the methamphetamine abuser with protracted abstinence (from Volkow et al., 2001, with permission)

Reneman and colleagues (2001b) compared cortical [^{123}I]β-CIT labelled SERT densities in different groups of MDMA users: twenty-two recent MDMA users who did not use MDMA for at least 3 weeks, 16 ex-MDMA users who had stopped using MDMA for more than 1 year, and 13 controls who claimed never to have used MDMA were enrolled. In addition, memory was assessed using a word recall test (Rey Aditory Verbal Learning Test). These are the same subjects as in an earlier study (Reneman et al., 2001a), with exception of the moderate MDMA users. Reduced cortical SERT densities were observed in recent, but not ex-MDMA users. However, both recent as well as ex-MDMA users recalled significantly less words compared to controls. Greater use of MDMA was associated with greater impairment in immediate verbal memory. However, memory performance was not associated with [^{123}I]β-CIT binding to cortical 5-HT transporters. A similar observation was made by Semple (1999), although in the Semple study MDMA users and non-users did not differ in neuropsychological performance. In contrast, Reneman (2000a) observed a strong association between post-synaptic 5-HT$_2$-receptor densities and memory performance. These findings may suggest that while the neurotoxic effects of MDMA on 5-HT neurones in the human cortex may be reversible, the effects of MDMA on memory function may be long(er) lasting. It An alternative explanation may be that cognitive abnormalities in MDMA users are not related to 5-HT neurotoxicity, but rather DA-neurotoxicity (Ricaurte et al., 2002).

Finally, one other study has investigated the relation between brain damage and memory function (Reneman et al., 2001c). Again, RAVLT was used to study 8 abstinent MDMA users and 7 controls. In addition ^{1}H-MRS was used in different brain regions of all MDMA users to measure NAA/Cr ratios. MDMA users recalled significantly less words compared to controls. In MDMA users, delayed memory function was strongly associated with NAA/Cr only in the prefrontal cortex, suggesting that greater decrements in memory function predicted lower NAA/Cr levels -and by inference greater neuronal dysfunction- in the prefrontal cortex of MDMA users.

Although most of these studies were conducted using small sample sizes with overlapping samples, they at least suggest an intriguing relationship between markers of brain damage and memory performance in MDMA users. However, they need be confirmed in a larger number of subjects.

Other amphetamine analogues currently used recreationally

In view of the fact that the number of potential synthetic amphetamine analogues that can be made and distributed are unlimited, only some can be discussed in this paper. The World Health Organization (2001) recently recommended for international control of the following analogues: 4-bromo-2,5-dimethoxyphenethylamine (2C-B), 4-methylthioamphetamine (4-MTA), and N-methyl-1-(1,3-benzodioxol 5-yl) 2-butamine (MBDB), only the neurotoxic effects of 4-MTA and MBDB on brain 5-HT and DA neurones have been studied in animals. Administration of an acute dose of 4-MTA did not affect

5-HT and 5-HIAA levels (Huang et al., 1992), suggesting that it has no 5-HT neurotoxic effects in rats. In contrast, MBDB, following a regimen of twice daily dosing for four days, produced significant decreases in 5-HT, 5-HIAA and [^{3}H]-paroxetine binding sites, although slightly less than MDMA. These data suggest that MBDB is a 5-HT neurotoxin, but may be less neurotoxic than MDMA (Johnson and Nichols, 1989).

Other amphetamine analogues that have been synthesized and used by humans are: para-methoxymethamphetamine (PMMA) and para-methoxyamphetamine (PMA). Both PMMA and PMA (80 mg/kg) have shown to produce comparable depletions of 5-HT, but these depletions are not as pronounced as those induced by a lower dose of MDMA (20 mg/kg), suggesting that PMMA and PMA are less potent than MDMA as a 5-HT neurotoxin (Steele et al., 1992). Striatal dopamine levels were unaffected by PMMA and PMA. On the other hand, 2,5-dimethoxy-4-methylamphetamine (DOM) does not cause significant loss of 5-HT uptake sites (McKenna et al., 1991). Neurotoxic effects of 4-bromo-2,5-dimethoxyamphetamine (DOB) have not been studied in animals.

5-HT neurotoxicity of none of the above mentioned analogues has been studied in humans.

Methamphetamine

Methamphetamine was first produced in the beginning of the 20th century by *N*-methyl substitution of amphetamine. Methamphetamine is a highly addictive drug (Woolverton et al., 1984), and its abuse has risen substantially. In several areas of the US one form of methamphetamine, crystal methamphetamine or "ice" grew in popularity in the 1980s. Its popularity declined again for a long period of time (0.4% in 1992), rising up again to 1.5% in 2001, an increase of 275% in the past decade (Johnston et al., 2002). The drug has now also become increasingly popular in Asian countries (Ahmad, 2002). In contrast, the average consumption of methamphetamines is still very limited in the EU (EMCDDA, 2001).

Animal studies

Methamphetamine administration to animals has been shown to produce long-lasting damage to DA and 5-HT neurones in animals (Koda and Gibb, 1973; Seiden et al., 1976; Bakhit et al., 1981; Ricaurte et al., 1980). After administration of methamphetamine animals develop long-lasting decreases in DA and 5-HT as well as their transporters (Seiden et al., 1976; Villemagne et al., 1998; Wagner et al., 1980). Although previous studies proposed that methamphetamine-induced DAT losses reflected irreversible terminal degeneration (Ricaurte and McCann, 1992b), recent studies in rodents (Friedman et al., 1998; Cass and Manning, 1999) and in nonhuman primates (Melega et al., 1997; Harvey et al., 2000) have revealed significant recovery with protracted abstinence. There is also evidence that methamphetamine affects nonmonoaminergic cortical neurones (Commins and Seiden, 1986; Ryan et al., 1990).

Human studies

PET

Recently a number of imaging studies have reported on the effects of methamphetamine on DA neurones in the human brain. To my knowledge, SERT densities have up until now not been studied. Using PET, reductions in DAT have been demonstrated in human methamphetamine users using the DAT ligands [^{11}C]WIN-35,248 and [^{11}C]*d-threo*-methylphenidate (McCann et al., 1998b; Volkow et al., 2001a; Sekine et al., 2001). DAT losses varied from 24 to 30% in these studies.

Linking biological markers of neuronal injury with behavioural function. Because significant reductions in DAT occur both with age (6–7% per decade for the 20–80 year age span) (Volkow et al., 1996) a concern arises as to whether methamphetamine abusers will place them at risk for Parkinsonism as they age. Although the DAT loss reported in methamphetamine abusers is smaller than that reported in Parkinson's disease (36 and 71%) (Frost et al., 1993), it is nonetheless associated with reduced motor speed and impaired verbal learning (Volkow et al., 2001a) and the severity of persistent psychiatric symptoms (Sekine et al., 2001).

Because potential risk for Parkinsonism and cognitive decline in methamphetamine users likely depends in part on the reversibility of the changes induced by methamphetamine, Volkow and colleagues (2001b) recently investigated whether DAT losses in methamphetamine abusers recover with protracted abstinence. Brain DAT densities as obtained with [^{11}C]*d-threo*-methylphenidate PET in 5 methamphetamine abusers during short abstinence (6 months) were retested during protracted abstinence (12–17 months). Significant increases in DAT were observed with protracted abstinence, suggesting that DA terminals recover after methamphetamine-induced damage or that DAT losses short after methamphetamine reflect temporary adaptive changes (i.e., downregulation or internalisation). Because recovery of DAT after methamphetamine treatment in animals takes longer (6–9 months) than if they were due to DAT downregulation or internalisation, the authors concluded that likely DAT losses recover in methamphetamine users. However, a parallel improvement in function was not observed, since neuropsychological function did not recover with protracted abstinence, in concordance with a similar study in MDMA users (Reneman et al., 2001b).

^{1}H MR Spectroscopy

One study has investigated NAA levels in 26 abstinent amphetamine users (Ernst et al., 2000) and 24 healthy subjects without a history of drug abuse.

Methamphetamine subjects were scanned after last use of the drug more than 2 weeks earlier. In the basal ganglia and frontal white matter NAA levels were significantly reduced in methamphetamine users compared to controls, suggestive of neuronal damage in abstinent methamphetamine users. Frontal white matter NAA levels correlated inversely with previous extent of methamphetamine use. The methamphetamine users also showed significantly reduced total creatine in the basal ganglia and increased choline-containing compounds, as well as MI in the frontal grey matter.

Amphetamine

The parent compound of the above described analogues, amphetamine (alpha-methyl-phen-methylamine), is a synthetic stimulant first produced in 1887. It has been used clinically to treat diseases such as mild depression and abnormally hyperactive children. The drug can cause psychological dependence and is often sold and used illegally. Although illicit drug use of amphetamine is limited in the US, Scandinavian countries are the main market for injected amphetamine and the UK for non-injected amphetamine (EMCDDA, 2001). The highest consumption of amphetamine in EU is found in the UK (EMCDDA, 2001).

Animal studies

Amphetamine has been shown to be neurotoxic to DA neurones in animals. Administration of amphetamine to animals, including non-human primates, results in decreases in DA levels and DAT densities (Melega et al., 1996; Steranka, 1983; Steranka et al., 1980). PET studies in amphetamine treated monkeys have shown reductions in striatal [^{18}F]fluoro-L-DOPA uptake in vervet monkeys (Melega et al., 1997, 1996). Furthermore, studies on rat striatal DA system have established that chronic amphetamine exposure results in neurotoxicity characterised by swollen nerve terminals and degenerated axons (Ridley et al., 1982; Ryan et al., 1990).

Human studies

SPECT

At present only one imaging study has been conducted to study the effects of amphetamine on DA neurones in humans. Using [^{123}I]β-CIT SPECT, Reneman and colleagues (2002c) recently reported reduced striatal DAT densities (−20%) in 9 combined MDMA and amphetamine use when compared with 29 sole MDMA users, after adjustment for age. Subjects were scanned after an abstention period of at least 3 weeks. The effects of MDMA on DAT density were also investigated in this study, as discussed previously. These initial observations in humans suggest that the intentional use of amphetamine by regular users of MDMA is associated with a reduction in nigrostriatal DA neurones.

Discussion and future studies

The goal of this article was to review available neuroimaging data in humans on 5-HT and DA neurotoxic effects of amphetamine analogues in humans, in addition to the parent compounds amphetamine and methamphetamine.

Of all amphetamine analogues, only the effects of MDMA and methamphetamine have been studied in human users. The reviewed neuroimaging studies provide suggestive evidence that users of MDMA are susceptible to 5-HT, but not DA neuronal damage, in which females may be more susceptible than males. The effects seem to be dose-related, possibly leading to functional impairments such as memory loss, reversible in some, but not all, brain regions. These results raise important questions as to the safety of MDMA by recreational users of this drug. However, before the findings of the presented studies can be validly used in prevention messages and clinical decision making, some of the results will have to be (re)confirmed in secondary studies, particularly concerning gender differences and (ir-) reversibility of MDMA's neurotoxic effects. In addition, neuroimaging reports suggest that users of amphetamine and methamphetamine may be at risk of developing reversible DA neurotoxicity, leading to long-term functional impairments such as reduced motor speed and impaired memory function. The effects of methamphetamine on 5-HT neurones have not been studied in the human brain.

Clearly, there are important methodological problems in studies conducted in humans, which are subject to ethical and methodological constraints (Curran, 2000; Kish, 2002). Consequently, until now most studies conducted in humans have had a retrospective design, in which evidence is indirect and differs in the degree to which any causative links can be implied between designer drugs use and neurotoxicity. To definitively establish a causative link between observed neurotoxic changes and MDMA-, or (meth)amphetamine use, an experimental study design would be needed. Therefore, at this moment, it cannot be ascertained that humans are susceptible to MDMA-induced 5-HT injury or (meth)amphetamine-induced DA-injury. One possible approach would be to assess people both before and after they took the drug. Neuroimaging techniques may be very helpful in providing such longitudinal studies in human drug users.

Whereas both PET and SPECT have proven to be useful techniques in assessing the potential risk of MDMA and related drugs, more recently introduced MR imaging tools hold great promise (Reneman, 2001d), but will yet have to prove their potential to the field. Currently available radioligands may not have the requisite sensitivity to detect smaller neurotoxic lesions. Without doubt more selective radioligands for SERTs will be developed for PET or SPECT in the future that may be more sensitive in detecting SERT reductions. Although none of the currently available techniques is perfect, converging lines of evidence are needed (using combinations of different imaging

Table 1. Summary of neuroimaging studies investigating potential neurotoxic effects of amphetamine analogues and parent compounds in the human brain

Investigating	Biological marker	Technique used	Reference
MDMA			
Neuronal loss	SERT	[^{11}C]McN5652 PET	McCann (1998a)
		[^{123}I]β-CIT SPECT	Semple (1999), Reneman (2001a,b)
	DAT	[^{123}I]β-CIT SPECT	Reneman (2002c)
	NAA	^{1}H-MRS	Chang (1999)
Liking neuronal injury with functional impairment	5-HT transporter + memory	[^{123}I]β-CIT SPECT	Reneman (2001b)
	NAA + memory	^{1}H-MRS	Reneman (2002b)
Amphetamine			
Neuronal loss	DAT	[^{123}I]β-CIT SPECT	Reneman (2002c)
Methamphetamine			
Neuronal loss	DAT	[^{11}C]WIN-35,248 PET	McCann et al. (1998b)
			Sekine et al. (2001)
		[^{11}C]*d-threo*-methylphenidate	Volkow et al. (2001a,b)
Liking neuronal injury with functional impairment	DAT + motor speed and memory	[^{11}C]*d-threo*-methylphenidate	Volkow et al. (2001a)
	DAT + psychiatric symptoms	[^{11}C]WIN-35,248 PET	Sekine et al. (2001)

techniques) to make an adequate risk assessment of MDMA and related rugs. In any case, the currently available preliminary data obtained using these methods can be strengthened considerably by laying the groundwork with preclinical studies in animals where direct, post-mortem neurochemical and neuroanatomical studies can be conducted.

Future studies will have to find out whether neurotoxic effects in heavy MDMA users tested to date also occur in less frequent users. Some have argued that even a single dose of MDMA may be neurotoxic in human beings (Gijsman et al., 1999; McCann and Ricaurte, 2001). MDMA users may be studied prospectively to shed light on the fate of damaged 5-HT neurones with age, and whether dysfunction (e.g., memory loss) resolves with abstinence or increases with age. More studies should be conducted combining neuroimaging studies with neuropsychological assessments to study links between brain damage and memory loss. In addition, more studies should be conducted focusing on other systems than the serotonergic system to increase our understanding on the effects of MDMA and subsequent compensatory mechanisms in the brain. Finally, as pointed out previously, because users of amphetamine analogues are typically polydrug users, it will be important to assess drug-drug interactions in animals. It may well be that one drug enhances the potential neurotoxicity of another drug used at a later time (Hegadoren et al., 1999).

If indeed amphetamine analogues and (meth)amphetamine lead to 5-HT and/or DA neuronal injury the health implications may be considerable, in which they will be responsible for early or late neuropsychiatric morbidity. Neuroimaging techniques will greatly contribute to our understanding of amphetamine analogue's short- and long-term effects in the human brain. The fact that all these techniques are non-invasive and most of them can be used repeatedly in the same subject is a very critical feature.

In conclusion, based on animal data and suggestive evidence in humans, it seems likely that MDMA is neurotoxic to brain 5-HT neurones and (meth)amphetamine to brain DA neurones, resulting in long-lasting functional impairments such as memory loss. Although very little is known about the effects of other amphetamine analogues, there are important questions as to the safety of these designer drugs to the human brain, in view of the fact that they are chemically closely related to MDMA and (meth)amphetamine.

References

Ahmad K (2002) Increased use of amphetamine-type stimulants threatens east Asian countries. Lancet 359: 1927

Backstrom I, Bergstrom M, Marcusson J (1989) High affinity [3H]paroxetine binding to serotonin uptake sites in human brain tissue. Brain Res 486: 261–268

Bakhit C, Morgan ME, Peat MA, Gibb JW (1981) Long-term effects of methamphetamine on the synthesis and metabolism of 5-hydroxytryptamine in various regions of the rat brain. Neuropharmacology 20: 1135–1140

Battaglia G, Yeh SY, O'Hearn E, Molliver ME, Kuhar MJ, De Souza EB (1987) 3,4-Methylenedioxymethamphetamine and 3,4-methylenedioxyamphetamine destroy serotonin terminals in rat brain: quantification of neurodegeneration by measurement of [^{3}H]paroxetine-labeled serotonin uptake sites. J Pharmacol Exp Ther 242: 911–916

Battaglia G, Yeh SY, De Souza EB (1988) MDMA-induced neurotoxicity: parameters of degeneration and recovery of brain serotonin neurons. Pharmacol Biochem Behav 29: 269–274

Boja JW, Patel A, Carroll FI, Rahman MA, Philip A, Lewin AH, Kopajtic TA, Kuhar MJ (1991) [^{125}I]RTI-55: a potent ligand for dopamine transporters. Eur J Pharmacol 194: 133–134

Boja JW, McNeill RM, Lewin AH, Abraham P, Carroll FI, Kuhar MJ (1992) Selective dopamine transporter inhibition by cocaine analogs. Neuroreport 3: 984–986

Cass WA, Manning MW (1999) Recovery of presynaptic dopaminergic functioning in rats treated with neurotoxic doses of methamphetamine. J Neurosci 19: 7653–7660

Chang L, Ernst T, Grob CS, Poland RE (1999) Cerebral ^{1}H MRS alterations in recreational 3,4-methylenedioxymethamphetamine (MDMA, "ecstasy") users. J Magn Reson Imaging 10: 521–526

Commins DL, Seiden LS (1986) alpha-Methyltyrosine blocks methylamphetamine-induced degeneration in the rat somatosensory cortex. Brain Res 365: 15–20

Commins DL, Vosmer G, Virus RM, Woolverton WL, Schuster CR, Seiden, LS (1987) Biochemical and histological evidence that methylenedioxymethylamphetamine (MDMA) is toxic to neurons in the rat brain. J Pharmacol Exp Ther 241: 338–345

Curran HV (2000) Is MDMA ('Ecstasy') neurotoxic in humans? An overview of evdience and of methodological problems in research. Neuropsychobiology 42: 34–41

EMCDDA (2001) Annual report on the state of the drugs problem in the European Union. http://annualreport.emcdda.org/multimedia/Annual_Report_2001/ar01_en.pdf

Ernst T, Chang L, Leonido-Yee M, Speck O (2000) Evidence for long-term neurotoxicity associated with methamphetamine abuse: a 1H MRS study. Neurology 54: 1344–1349

Farde L, Halldin C, Muller L, Suhara T, Karlsson P, Hall H (1994) PET study of [^{11}C]β-CIT binding to monoamine transporters in the monkey and human brain. Synapse 16: 93–103

Friedman SD, Castaneda E, Hodge GK (1998) Long-term monoamine depletion, differential recovery, and subtle behavioral impairment following methamphetamine-induced neurotoxicity. Pharmacol Biochem Behav 61: 35–44

Frost JJ, Rosier AJ, Reich SG, Smith JS, Ehlers MD, Snyder SH, Ravert HT, Dannals RF (1993) Positron emission tomographic imaging of the dopamine transporter with 11C-WIN 35,428 reveals marked declines in mild Parkinson's disease. Ann Neurol 34: 423–431

Gibb JW, Stone DM, Stahl DC, Hanson GR (1987) The effects of amphetamine-like designer drugs on monoaminergic systems in rat brain. NIDA Res Monogr 76: 316–321

Gijsman HJ, Verkes RJ, van Gerven JMA, Cohen AF (1999) MDMA study. Neuropsychopharmacology 21: 597

Gurevich EV, Joyce JN (1996) Comparison of [^{3}H]paroxetine and [^{3}H]cyanoimipramine for quantitative measurement of serotonin transporter sites in human brain. Neuropsychopharmacology 14: 309–323

Harvey DC, Lacan G, Tanious SP, Melega WP (2000) Recovery from methamphetamine induced long-term nigrostriatal dopaminergic deficits without substantia nigra cell loss. Brain Res 871: 259–270

Hatzidimitriou G, McCann UD, Ricaurte GA (1999) Altered serotonin innervation patterns in the forebrain of monkeys treated with (+/−)3,4-methylenedioxymethamphetamine seven years previously: factors influencing abnormal recovery. J Neurosci 19: 5096–5107

Hegadoren KM, Baker GB, Bourin M (1999) 3,4-Methylenedioxy analogues of amphetamine: defining the risks to humans. Neurosci Biobehav Rev 23: 539–553

Higuchi T, Graham SH, Fernandez EJ, Rooney WD, Gaspary HL, Weiner MW, Maudsley AA (1997) Effects of severe global ischemia on N-acetylaspartate and other metabolites in the rat brain. Magn Reson Med 37: 851–857

Howe FA, Maxwell RJ, Saunders DE, Brown MM, Griffiths JR (1993) Proton spectroscopy in vivo. Magn Reson Q 9: 31–59

Huang X, Marona-Lewicka D, Nichols DE (1992) p-methylthioamphetamine is a potent new non-neurotoxic serotonin-releasing agent. Eur J Pharmacol 229: 31–38

Johnson MP, Hoffman AJ, Nichols DE (1986) Effects of the enantiomers of MDA, MDMA and related analogues on [^{3}H]serotonin and [^{3}H]dopamine release from superfused rat brain slices. Eur J Pharmacol 132: 269–276

Johnston LD, O'Malley PM, Bachman JG (2002) Monitoring the future national results on adolescent drug use: overview of key findings, 2001. National Institute of Drug Abuse, Bethesda, MD (NIH Pub. No. 02-5105)

Kamien JB, Johanson CE, Schuster CR, Woolverton WL (1986) The effects of (+/−)-methylenedioxymethamphetamine and (+/−)-methylenedioxyamphetamine in monkeys trained to discriminate (+)-amphetamine from saline. Drug Alcohol Depend 18: 139–147

Kieven MS, Seiden LS (1992) Methamphetamine-induced neurotoxicity: structure activity relationships. Ann NY Acad Sci 654: 292–301

Kish SJ (2002) How strong is the evidence that brain serotonin neurons are damaged in human users of ecstasy? Pharmacol Biochem Behav 71: 845–855

Koda LY, Gibb JW (1973) Adrenal and striatal tyrosine hydroxylase activity after methamphetamine. J Pharmacol Exp Ther 185: 42–48

Kuikka JT, Tiihonen J, Bergstrom KA, Karhu J, Hartikainen P, Viinamaki H, Lansimies E, Lehtonen J, Hakola P (1995) Imaging of serotonin and dopamine transporters in the living human brain. Eur J Nucl Med 22: 346–350

Laruelle M, Baldwin RM, Malison RT, Zea-Ponce Y, Zoghbi SS, al-Tikriti MS, Sybirska EH, Zimmermann RC, Wisniewski G, Neumeyer JL (1993) SPECT imaging of dopamine and serotonin transporters with [^{123}I]β-CIT: pharmacological characterization of brain uptake in nonhuman primates. Synapse 13: 295–309

Lew R, Sabol KE, Chou C, Vosmer GL, Richards J, Seiden LS (1996) Methylenedioxymethamphetamine-induced serotonin deficits are followed by partial recovery over a 52-week period, part II. Radioligand binding and autoradiography studies. J Pharmacol Exp Ther 276: 855–865

Melega WP, Quintana J, Raleigh MJ, Stout DB, Yu DC, Lin KP, Huang SC, Phelps ME (1996) 6-[^{18}F]fluoro-L-DOPA-PET studies show partial reversibility of long-term effects of chronic amphetamine in monkeys. Synapse 22: 63–69

Melega WP, Raleigh MJ, Stout DB, Lacan G, Huang SC, Phelps ME (1997) Recovery of striatal dopamine function after acute amphetamine- and methamphetamine-induced neurotoxicity in the vervet monkey. Brain Res 766: 113–120

McCann UD, Ricaurte GA (2001) Caveat emptor: editors beware. Neuropsychopharmacology 24: 333–334

McCann UD, Szabo Z, Scheffel U, Dannals RF, Ricaurte GA (1998a) Positron emission tomographic evidence of toxic effect of MDMA ("Ecstasy") on brain serotonin neurones in human beings. Lancet 352: 1433–1437

McCann UD, Wong DF, Yokoi F, Villemagne V, Dannals RF, Ricaurte GA (1998b) Reduced striatal dopamine transporter density in abstinent methamphetamine and methcathinone users: evidence from positron emission tomography studies with [^{11}C]WIN-35,428. J Neurosci 18: 8417–8422

McKenna DJ, Guan XM, Shulgin AT (1991) 3,4-Methylenedioxyamphetamine (MDA) analogues exhibit differential effects on synaptosomal release of 3H-dopamine and 3H-5-hydroxytryptamine. Pharmacol Biochem Behav 38: 505–512

Molliver ME, Berger UV, Mamounas LA, Molliver DC, O'Hearn E, Wilson, MA (1990) Neurotoxicity of MDMA and related compounds: anatomic studies. Ann NY Acad Sci 600: 649–661

Mordenti J, Chappell (1989) The use of interspecies scaling in toxicokinetics. In: Yacobi A, Kelly J, Batra V (eds) Toxicokinetics and new drug development. Pergamon Press, New York, pp 42–96

Obergriesser T, Ende G, Braus DF, Henn FA (2001) Hippocampal ^{1}H-MRSI in ecstasy users. Eur Arch Psychiatry Clin Neurosci 251: 114–116

O'Hearn E, Battaglia G, De Souza EB, Kuhar MJ, Molliver ME (1988) Methylenedioxyamphetamine (MDA) and methylenedioxymethamphetamine (MDMA) cause selective ablation of serotonergic axon terminals in forebrain: immunocytochemical evidence for neurotoxicity. J Neurosci 8: 2788–2803

Parrott AC (2000) Human research on MDMA (3,4-methylenedioxymethamphetamine) neurotoxicity: cognitive and behavioural indices of change. Neuropsychobiology 42: 17–24

Parsey RV, Kegeles LS, Hwang DR, Simpson N, Abi-Dargham A, Mawlawi O, Slifstein M, Van Heertum RL, Mann JJ, Laruelle M (2000) In vivo quantification of brain serotonin transporters in humans using [^{11}C]McN 5652. J Nucl Med 41: 1465–1477

Pirker W, Asenbaum S, Hauk M, Kandlhofer S, Tauascher J, Willeit M, Neurmeister A, Praschak-Rieder N, Angelberger P, Brücke T (2000) Imaging serotonin and dopamine transporters with ^{123}I-β-CIT SPECT: binding kinetics and effects of normal aging. J Nucl Med 41: 36–44

Pope HG Jr, Ionescu-Pioggia M, Pope KW (2001) Drug use and life style among college undergraduates: a 30-year longitudinal study. Am J Psychiatry 158: 1519–1521

Reneman L, Booij J, Schmand B, van den Brink W, Gunning B (2000a) Memory disturbances in "Ecstasy" users are correlated with an altered brain serotonin neurotransmission. Psychopharmacology 148: 322–324

Reneman L, Booij J, de Bruin K, de Wolff FA, Gunning WB, den Heeten GJ, vd Brink W (2001a) Effects of dose, sex, and long-term abstention from use on toxic effects of MDMA (ecstasy) on brain serotonin neurons. Lancet 358: 1864–1869

Reneman L, Lavalaye J, Booij J, Schmand B, de Wolff FA, vd Brink W, den Heeten GJ, Booij J (2001b) Cortical serotonin transporter density and verbal memory in individuals who stopped using 3,4-methylenedioxymethaphetamine (MDMA or "Ecstasy") — preliminary findings. Arch Gen Psychiatry 58: 901–906

Reneman L, Majoie CBLM, Schmand B, vd Brink W, den Heeten GJ (2001c) Prefrontal N-acetylaspartate is strongly associated with memory performance in (abstinent) Ecstasy users: preliminary report. Biol Psychiatry 50: 550–554

Reneman L, Majoie CBLM, Habraken JBA, den Heeten GJ (2001d) Diffusion and the effects of Ecstasy (MDMA) on the brain in abstinent users: initial observations with diffusion and perfusion MR imaging. Radiology 220: 611–617

Reneman L, Booij J, Habraken JBA, de Bruin K, Hatzidimitriou G, den Heeten GJ, Ricaurte GA (2002a) Validity of [^{123}I]β-CIT SPECT in detecting MDMA-induced serotonergic neurotoxicity. Synapse 46: 199–205

Reneman L, Majoie CBLM, Flick H, den Heeten GJ (2002b) Reduced N-acetylaspartate levels in the frontal cortex of 3,4-methylenedioxymethaphetamine ("Ecstasy") users — preliminary results. AJNR Am J Neuroradiol 23: 231–237

Reneman L, Booij J, Lavalaye J, de Bruin K, Reitsma JB, Gunning WB, den Heeten GJ, van den Brink W (2002c) Use of amphetamine by recreational users of ecstasy is associated with reduced striatal dopamine transporter densities: a [^{123}I]β-CIT SPECT study. Psychopharmacology 159: 335–340

Ricaurte GA, McCann UD (1992b) Neurotoxic amphetamine analogues: effects in monkeys and implications for humans. Ann NY Acad Sci 648: 371–382

Ricaurte GA, Schuster CR, Seiden LS (1980) Long-term effects of repeated methylamphetamine administration on dopamine and serotonin neurons in the rat brain: a regional study. Brain Res 193: 153–163

Ricaurte G, Bryan G, Strauss L, Seiden L, Schuster C (1985) Hallucinogenic amphetamine selectively destroys brain serotonin nerve terminals. Science 229: 986–988

Ricaurte GA, DeLanney LE, Irwin I, Langston JW (1988) Toxic effects of MDMA on central serotonergic neurones in the primate: importance of route and frequency of drug administration. Brain Res 446: 165–168

Ricaurte GA, Martello AL, Katz JL, Martello MB (1992a) Lasting effects of (+/−)-3,4-methylenedioxymethamphetamine (MDMA) on central serotonergic neurons in non-human primates: neurochemical observations. J Pharmacol Exp Ther 261: 616–622

Ricaurte GA, Yuan J, McCann UD (2000) (+/−)3,4-Methylenedioxymethamphetamine ("Ecstasy")-induced serotonin neurotoxicity: studies in animals. Neuropsychobiology 42: 5–10

Ricaurte GA, Yuan J, Hatzidimitriou G, Cord BJ, McCann UD (2002) Severe dopaminergic neurotoxicity in primates after a common recreational dose regimen of MDMA ("ecstasy"). Science 297: 2260–2263

Ridley RM, Baker HF, Owen F, Cross AJ, Crow TJ (1982) Behavioural and biochemical effects of chronic amphetamine treatment in the vervet monkey. Psychopharmacology 78: 245–251

Ryan LJ, Linder JC, Martone ME, Groves PM (1990) Histological and ultrastructural evidence that D-amphetamine causes degeneration in neostriatum and frontal cortex of rats. Brain Res 518: 67–77

Scanzello CR, Hatzidimitriou G, Martello AL, Katz JL, Ricaurte GA (1993) Serotonergic recovery after (+/−)3,4-(methylenedioxy) methamphetamine injury: observations in rats. J Pharmacol Exp Ther 264: 1484–1491

Scheffel U, Ricaurte GA (1990) Paroxetine as an in vivo indicator of 3,4-methylenedioxymethamphetamine neurotoxicity: a presynaptic serotonergic positron emission tomograpy ligand? Brain Res 527: 89–95

Scheffel U, Dannals RF, Cline EJ, Ricaurte GA, Carroll FI, Abraham P, Lewin AH, Kuhar MJ (1992) [$^{123/125}$I]RTI-55, an in vivo label for the serotonin transporter. Synapse 11: 134–139

Scheffel U, Szabo Z, Mathews WB, Finley PA, Dannals RF, Ravert HT, Szabo K, Yuan J, Ricaurte GA (1998) In vivo detection of short- and long-term MDMA neurotoxicity–a positron emission tomography study in the living baboon brain. Synapse 29: 183–192

Schifano F, Di Furia L, Forza G, Minicuci N, Bricolo R (1998) MDMA ('ecstasy') consumption in the context of polydrug abuse: a report on 150 patients. Drug Alcohol Depend 52: 85–90

Schmidt CJ (1987a) Neurotoxicity of the psychedelic amphetamine, methylenedioxymethamphetamine. J Pharmacol Exp Ther 240: 1–7

Schmidt CJ, Taylor VL (1987b) Depression of rat brain tryptophan hydroxylase activity following the acute administration of methylenedioxymethamphetamine. Biochem Pharmacol 36: 4095–4102

Schmidt CJ, Wu L, Lovenberg W (1986) Methylenedioxymethamphetamine: a potentially neurotoxic amphetamine analogue. Eur J Pharmacol 124: 175–178

Seiden LS, Fischman MW, Schuster CR (1976) Long-term methamphetamine induced changes in brain catecholamines in tolerant rhesus monkeys. Drug Alcohol Depend 1: 215–219

Sekine Y, Iyo M, Ouchi Y, Matsunaga T, Tsukada H, Okada H, Yoshikawa E, Fatutsubashi M, Takei N, Mori N (2001) Methamphetamine-related psychiatric symptoms and reduced brain dopamine transporters studied with PET. Am J Psychiatry 158: 1206–1214

Semple DM, Ebmeier KP, Glabus MF, O'Carroll RE, Johnstone EC (1999) Reduced in vivo binding to the serotonin transporter in the cerebral cortex of MDMA ('ecstasy') users. Br J Psychiatry 175: 63–69

Shulgin A, Shulgin A (1991) Pihkal: a chemical love story. Transform Press, Berkeley, CA

Steele TD, Katz JL, Ricaurte GA (1992) Evaluation of the neurotoxicity of N-methyl-1-(4-methoxyphenyl)-2-aminopropane (para-methoxymethamphetamine, PMMA). Brain Res 589: 349–352

Steele TD, McCann UD, Ricaurte GA (1994) 3,4-Methylenedioxymethamphetamine (MDMA, "Ecstasy"): pharmacology and toxicology in animals and humans. Addiction 89: 539–551

Steranka LR (1983) Long-term effects of a priming dose and short-term infusion of amphetamine on striatal dopamine neurones in rats. Eur J Pharmacol 96: 159–163

Steranka LR, Sanders-Bush E (1980) Long-term effects of continuous exposure to amphetamine on brain dopamine concentration and synaptosomal uptake in mice. Eur J Pharmacol 65: 439–443

Stone DM, Stahl DC, Hanson GR, Gibb JW (1986) The effects of 3,4-methylenedioxymethamphetamine (MDMA) and 3,4-methylenedioxyamphetamine (MDA) on monoaminergic systems in the rat brain. Eur J Pharmacol 128: 41–48

Stone DM, Johnson M, Hanson GR, Gibb JW (1987) A comparison of the neurotoxic potential of methylenedioxyamphetamine (MDA) and its N-methylated and N-ethylated derivatives. Eur J Pharmacol 134: 245–248

Strote J, Lee JE, Wechsler H (2002) Increasing MDMA use among college students: results of a national survey. J Adolesc Health 30: 64–72

Urenjak J, Williams SR, Gadian DG, Noble M (1993) Proton nuclear magnetic resonance spectroscopy unambiguously identifies different neural cell types. J Neurosci 13: 981–989

Villemagne V, Yuan J, Wong DF, Dannals RF, Hatzidimitriou G, Mathews, Ravert HT, Musachio J, McCann UD, Ricaurte GA (1998) Brain dopamine neurotoxicity in baboons treated with doses of methamphetamine comparable to those recreationally abused by humans: evidence from [^{11}C]WIN-35,428 positron emission tomography studies and direct in vitro determinations. J Neurosci 18: 419–427

Volkow ND, Ding YS, Fowler JS, Wang GJ, Logan J, Gatley SJ, Hitzemann R, Smith G, Fields SD, Gur R (1996) Dopamine transporters decrease with age. J Nucl Med 37: 554–559

Volkow ND, Chang L, Wang G, Fowler JS, Leonido-Yee M, Franceschi D, Sedler MJ, Gatley SJ, Hitzemann R, Ding YS, Logan J, Wong C, Miller EN (2001a) Association of dopamine transporter reduction with psychomotor impairment in methamphetamine abusers. Am J Psychiatry 158: 377–382

Volkow ND, Chang L, Wang GJ, Fowler JS, Franceschi D, Sedler M, Gatley SJ, Miller E, Hitzemann R, Ding YS, Logan J (2001b) Loss of dopamine transporters in methamphetamine abusers recovers with protracted abstinence. J Neurosci 21: 9414–9418

Wagner GC, Ricaurte GA, Seiden LS, Schuster CR, Miller RJ, Westley J (1980) Long-lasting depletions of striatal dopamine and loss of dopamine uptake sites following repeated administration of methamphetamine. Brain Res 81: 151–160

World Health Organization (2001) WHO Expert Committee on Drug Dependence. Thirty-second report. World Health Organ Tech Rep Ser 903: i–v, pp 1–26

Woolverton WL, Cervo L, Johanson CE (1984) Effects of repeated methamphetamine administration on methamphetamine self-adminsitration in rhesus monkeys. Pharmacol Biochem Behav 21: 737–741

Zhou FC, Tao-Cheng J, Segu L, Patel T, Wang Y (1998) Serotonin transporters are located on the axons beyond the synaptic junctions: anatomical and functional evidence. Brain Res 805: 241–254

Authors' address: L. Reneman, MD PhD, Department of Radiology, G1-214, Academic Medical Center, Meibergdreef 9, 1105 AZ Amsterdam, The Netherlands, e-mail: l.reneman@amc.uva.nl

Early intervention strategies in substance abuse

M. Kurz

Department of Psychiatry, Innsbruck University Hospital, Mutters, Austria

Summary. Since the mid-eighties many efforts have been made to develop spezialized intervention strategies and interview techniques aiming at harm reduction and motivational enhancement in patients with substance related disorders. Firstly, the "Transtheoretical Model of Change" by Prochaska and DiClemente, which defines motivation as a dynamic process with several stage dependent intervention possibilities. Secondly, the "Motivational Interviewing" technique by Miller and Rollnick, who strongly suggest an empathic communication style deriving from humanistic psychology. It has been shown that especially persons in early stages of substance related disorders profited very well from such early interventions. Psychiatric institutions not involved in specialized addiction treatment have to face frequent comorbid substance abuse among their patients. Findings of the efficacy of early interventions in general psychiatry are encouraging. Despite there is strong evidence of efficacy of early and motivational intervention strategies in several medical fields, their implementation tends to be very difficult.

Introduction

Disorders related to abuse or dependence from alcohol and other drugs are among the most widespread and serious disorders in medicine. The economic costs of substance abuse have been estimated to reach $ 428.1 billion in the U.S. in 1995 (Rice, 1999). The WHO and World Bank (Murray and Lopez, 1996) report alcohol abuse being responsible for 9.6% of all life years lost by disease, injury or death among developed countries.

Although we have a well developed health care system, most of the affected persons do not receive specific treatment. In Germany, a country with an enormous number of different in- and outpatient treatment facilites, only 2.5% of all alcohol dependent subjects undergo specific treatment per year, whereas 70% visit their general practitioner at least once a year and about 25% are seen as inpatients in non-psychiatric medical wards (Wienberg, 1995). This imbalance is also reported from other European countries and from the U.S. (Fleming, 2000).

One reason for the gap between primary health care, general psychiatry and substance abuse treatment facilities is the lack of knowledge about the special psychological processes and interaction styles among substance dependent or abusing subjects in basic medical and psychosocial education. Furthermore, specialized treatment facilities sometimes appear rigid and strange to many outside of these institutions with regard to interactions between professionals and patients. Certain habits, attitudes and jargons inside the alcohol and drug care systems are not very helpful in bridging the gap to the „outside world". There is also a negative selection of patients with more severe social, psychiatric and medical problems in specialized treatment units.

Especially problem drinkers or less severely dependent persons without comorbidity and with good social support do not seek specialized counseling or treatment because they do not suffer from any personal or social pressure to do so. These patients are the main target group of early intervention strategies. The prevention of further damage instead of waiting until the patients get sufficient motivation towards abstinence after having "hit the rock bottom" is the main goal here. Several studies have shown the effectiveness of early interventions in general medical and primary care settings (Kristensohn, 1983; Chick, 1991; Nilssen, 1991; Richmond, 1995; WHO, 1996; Fleming, 1997; Senft, 1997; Welte, 1998; Tomson, 1998).

Motivation: state or trait?

Early intervention strategies are adressed at patients who need a strengthening of intrinsic motivation to change their alcohol and drug use patterns and/or to seek specialized treatment if their substance-related problems need professional management. Over the last 15 years, the construct of motivation in addiction psychology has changed profoundly. In the past, most substance dependent persons were judged to suffer from low motivation as part of their diagnosis. Defense mechanisms like denial, rationalization and projection/externalization, which are very common in substance related disorders, seemed to strongly support this notion. This also provoked confrontational and sometimes devaluating therapeutic interaction styles which have been thought to be the best way to confront the patients and to break their denial and defense. As it is well known, this did not work, but just to be nice and understanding was not the solution either. Especially at the time of first contact, the patients see themselves confronted with the unthinkable and unbearable fact of being diagnosed as substance dependent. It is not difficult to understand that they cannot show sufficient motivation towards long-term abstinence or far-reaching changes in their lifestyles at this moment. If the physician interpretes this as an individual personality-based lack of motivation, the patient would likely retreat further treatment. Clinical experience and knowledge about the natural history of addictive disorders show that the development of motivation needs time and must be supported by positive social and interactional experiences.

What are strong motivators?

If one distinguishes between intrinsic and extrinsic motivational sources, it has been shown that intrinsic motivators are clearly stronger in terms of successfully maintaining behavioral changes and/or treatment effectiveness. A good example for intrinsic motivation is the positive acceptance of personal responsibility. External motivators are often necessary to start the process of change, i.e. short-term abstinence to avoid further negative social consequences. Social pressure is the most frequent motivator for patients to start treatment. Many substance abuse treatment units are mainly confronted with patients seeking treatment to avoid negative social consequences. Many of these patients did not have enough time in the course of their illness to develop intrinsic motivation (i.e. an internal belief that the problem is severe enough to deserve treatment) (Fleming, 2000). On the other hand, there is a positive correlation between problem severity and internal motivation to change drinking behavior (DiClemente, 1999), although heavier drinkers do not seek treatment more frequently than lighter drinkers.

The transtheoretical model of change

Motivation is a complex issue which seems to have a chronological, developmental and individual dynamic. Therefore the different goals of motivation will be subject to change correspondingly. Prochaska and DiClemente (1994) developed the stage model of change, defining motivation as a dynamic process with certain stages that can change over time and can be successfully supported even when motivation seems very low. The model of change was first developed for smokers. It can be used for many types of self-destructive behavior and has enormously improved the therapeutic repertoire of alcohol and drug treatment professionals.

The 6 steps are shown in Fig. 1. The development of change is thought to resemble a circle, where one enters at the stage of precontemplation, passes contemplation, preparation, reaches maintenance and (at least theoretically concerning substance dependence) moves forward to the circle exit at the termination stage.

Specific characteristics and treatment goals of the different stages are listed in Table 1.

At the precontemplation stage, patients do not feel any need to change their drug use, on the contrary, they report many positive aspects of drug use. Problematization, use of motivational strategies and the evaluation of practical needs and self-regulatory activities are the main professional issues at this stage.

Change becomes a possibility at the contemplation stage. The patients seek for specific information and show growing awareness of their ambivalence concerning drug use. Nevertheless they are not really prepared to take action soon. At this stage the professional has to support the decision making

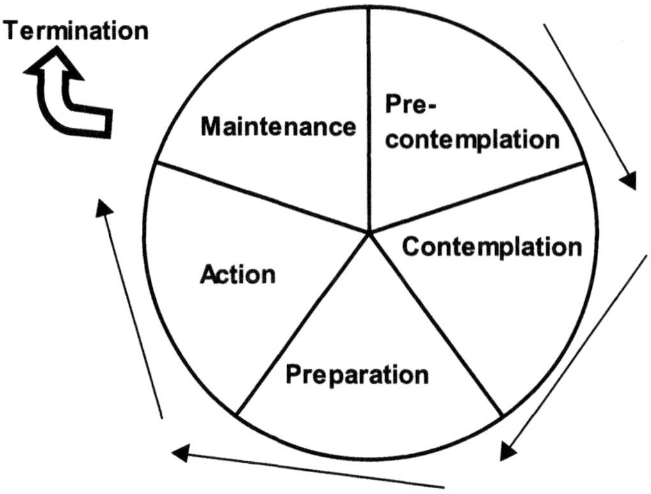

Fig. 1. Stages of change (Prochaska and DiClemente)

towards action, to raise the growing consciousness and to reevaluate self and environment of the patient.

Being at the preparation stage means the patients showing growing commitment to action and planning to take action soon. Sustained strengthening this commitment, but also helping the patient to set realistic goals and to develop a concrete change plan is important now.

Entering the action stage, the modifying of drug use becomes obvious and the patient starts to develop preventive skills by himself. The intervention contains further increasing self efficacy and offering behavioral change methods.

At the maintenance stage, patients show active efforts to maintain their new drug use behavior. The main topics at this stage are the reflection of difficult situations in daily life and further support in gaining self-efficacy.

Substance abuse treatment units are primarily adressing patients of the action stage. But as mentioned before, a large proportion of their patients are clearly contemplating or preparing.

Therefore they have a greater risk receiving inadequate therapy offered in specialized institutions. It could be argued that treatment failures (relapse, withdrawal, lack of efficacy) in specialized units are a consequence of inadequate motivational preparation for this mostly abstinence-oriented type of therapeutic intervention.

In general medical and psychiatric areas professionals are mostly confronted with patients in acute states of secondary illnesses deriving from abusive or dependent substance consumption. As the chief problem is drug consumption, classical medical intervention is clear: stop it and you will avoid further illness. Clinical experience shows that this statement is objectively correct but often fails to correspond to the actual needs and potentials of the patient, who will consequently often not follow this advice.

Table 1. Stages of change by Prochaska and DiClemente

	Patient characteristics	Intervention goals
Precontemplation	no need to change drug use in any way many positive aspects of drug use	problematization, use of motivational strategies evaluation of practical needs and self-regulatory activities
Contemplation	changing becomes a possibility information seeking awareness of ambivalence not prepared to change	enabling to a decision to act raising of consciousness reevaluation of self and environment
Preparation	growing commitment to action planning to take action soon	strengthen commitment set realistic goals, develop change plan
Action	overtly modifying of drug use development of preventive skills	increase self-efficacy and offer behavior change methods
Maintenance	active efforts to maintain changes	Reflection of difficult situations further support concerning self-efficacy

Modified from Connors et al. (2001)

Different goals of motivational efforts

Early intervention in substance dependent patients therefore has to focus on issues acceptable for the patient to be successful. It is helpful to differentiate the goals of motivation to be able to intervene adequately (Schwoon, 1998):

1. Motivation towards treatment. This is influenced by the subjective extent of the patients' suffering, the likelihood of success and the practicability of the treatment efforts (short term goal).
2. Motivation towards becoming and remaining abstinent or to change consumption style (medium/long-term goal).
3. Motivation towards lifestyle changes under new drug consumption conditions (long-term goal).

In the case of more severely dependent subjects, the main goal of early intervention is to start further specific treatment, whereas in abusing patients the main goal will be to return to a subjectively and objectively acceptable use of psychotropic substances.

Early intervention strategies

There are two well evaluated intervention techniques which have proved to be effective in different settings.

Brief intervention

This standardized intervention is mainly applied in primary health care or general medical contexts, where physicians and nurses do not have enough time for longer drug-specific interviews with patients. Brief intervention is based on 5 essential steps (Fleming, 1999):

— Assessment and direct feedback: The physician assesses the patient's alcohol or drug consumption together with other "hard facts" related to the substance misuse (i.e. liver dysfunction, hypertension, diarrhea, etc.) and confronts the patient with these facts in a concerned manner.

— Negotiation and goal setting: Physician and patient try to find an agreement concerning an individual goal of reduction of alcohol or drug use.

— Behavioral modification techniques: High-risk situations are identified and coping possibilities for their management are discussed. It is also important to show the patient ways of establishing a specific support network.

— Self-help-directed bibliotherapy: The patients receive information material on alcohol or drug use and related disorders together with suggestions for behavioral modification exercises.

— Follow-up and reinforcement: This is a very important part if interventions are to have sustained positive effects. The physician offers about 4 follow-up visits and opportunities for telephone support to the patient.

Clearly there are many opportunities to modify this intervention strategy depending on the local health care system. In countries with well established public alcohol and drug counseling and treatment facilities, the intervention goals could also include a visit in a specialized outpatient treatment unit, especially if the patient shows clear signs of dependent alcohol and/or drug consumption.

Fleming (1999) distinguishes between three types of background variables with different intervention goals, where brief intervention can be helpful. Firstly, a reduction of substance consumption in samples at risk for health consequences in general. Secondly, the improvement of compliance and a support of abstinence in patients with comorbid disorders and psychopharmacotherapy. Thirdly, enabling alcohol-dependent patients to seek specialized treatment. Brief intervention has proved to be effective in all these indications (Fleming, 1999).

Motivational interviewing (MI)

The motivational interviewing technique was developed by Miller and Rollnick (1991, 2002). It is adressed to professionals dealing with many different self-destructive behavioral problems (smoking, overeating, etc.) and is widely used in the fields of addiction counseling and treatment.

Overall, motivational interviewing consists of two chronological steps: In phase 1, the main goal is to build motivation for change, in phase 2, when clear signs of enhanced motivation and readiness for change arise, efforts shift to strengthening the patient's commitment to change.

MI builds up collaboration with the patient by using the patient's experience and perspective rather by confrontation with "objective reality". In early stages of awareness of the disorder MI emphasizes on evocating intrinsic motivation which is presumed to be the patients' own resource. Common interaction strategies are more educational and look for the patients' deficits to improve them with external help.

The medical profession is very often socialized in a authoritarian and hierarchical way. Therefore patients are expected to follow a physician's advice. MI lets the patient find his own solutions and goals even if these are not in line with the physicians' perspective.

However, MI is not just empathic listening; it always pursues the goal of vigorously enabling the patient to change a self-destructive behavior.

Table 2 shows the four general principles of MI.

Even though MI respects the patients' decision in any instance, it is not a laissez-faire style of professional communication. It goes along with the patients' needs and abilities but at the same time directly targets at a concrete change of behavior.

Table 2. Principles of motivational interviewing

1.	Express Empathy	Acceptance and avoidance of labeling the patient Reflective listening, no judging, critizizing and blaming, effort to understand subjective perspective without agreeing or rejecting; Ambivalence is normal
2.	Develop Discrepancy	Amplify a discrepancy between present behavior and broader goals and values, so that change becomes important. The patient should present ideas and plans by himself
3.	Roll with Resistance	Avoidance of physicians' arguing in favor of change No direct opposition of resistance No imposition of perspectives by the physician Patients are free to decide what professional offers and opinions they can take or leave and are the primary resource in finding answers Emerging resistance should always be a signal for reflecting and changing ones communication style rather than insisting on the "truth"
4.	Support Self-Efficacy	Strengthening the patient's belief in the possibility of change is important for his ability to take acion towards change The patient and not the physician is responsible to carry out behavioral change The physican's own optimistic belief in the abilities of the patient can become a self-fulfilling prophecy

Modified from Miller and Rollnick (2002)

The efficacy of Motivational Interviewing and its adapted variations have been proven in the field of alcohol and drug related disorders. In a recently published review by Burke et al. (2002) it has been concluded that MI is more efficacious than no treatment, both as a stand-alone intervention and as prelude to other treatments. Patients with high degree of anger seem to profit most from MI interventions. The generalizability and the clinical significance of the studies on MI appear to be strong, despite of a weak methodology in some of the studies. We know little about the way how MI exerts his effects, research suggests that they seem to be strongly clinician-mediated.

Early intervention possibilities in general psychiatry

But there are not only non-psychiatric medical areas which have to deal with patients with a lack of awareness of their substance abuse problem.

Psychiatric patients often show a considerable concomitant abuse of psychotropic substances to improve their impaired emotional condition. This high-risk consumption behaviour often remains disregarded by psychiatric clinicians (Hansen, 2000) and is followed by lower access and treatment adherence to mental health care services and worsening of the primary disorder (Sithartan et al., 1999). Comorbidity among patients with substance related disorders like anxiety, depression or personality disorders are well known and tolerated to a certain extent in addiction treatment services. Patients with schizophrenia or bipolar disorder have been reported to suffer from substance related disorders in up to 50% (Regier et al., 2002). These patients with severe and chronic disorders as well as personality disorders with high emotional instability have serious problems to follow addiction related treatment concepts.

Integrated treatment approaches proved to be efficacious in patients with dual diagnoses, but also show high drop-out rates. Thus, enhancing the patients' long-term motivation is the major challenge.

There are three main goals of motivational interventions in patients with dual diagnoses (for detailed review see Handmaker et al., 2002).

Firstly, to ensure the patients' engagement in further treatment at the transition from in- to out-patient care. Motivational interviewing prior to discharge has been shown to lead to improved aftercare adherence (Handmaker, 2002).

Secondly, treatment adherence during out-patient care. There is strong agreement that this is one of the most important outcome criteria. Very few studies have been done, but there is evidence that specific motivational interventions favour the adherence to out-patient treatment including medication compliance and — in one case — the reduction of alcohol consumption.

In a recent study Baker et al. (2002) investigated the effects of motivational interviewing among psychiatric inpatients with substance use disorders. The authors found MI not to be more effective compared to no intervention in terms of further attendance of a specialist substance misuse service. The patient sample was dominated by chronic patients with several complications and secondary disorders. It is likely that these patients need more intensive interventions because they may not be able to recognize the goals of the interview due to their severe cognitive and social deficits.

Implementation of early intervention and motivational interviewing

Motivation enhancing strategies appear more effective when applied as opportunistic interventions in the general medical field or in psychiatric patients without a long history of unsuccessful substance abuse treatment.

As there is little empirical knowledge about the possibilities of early interventions in general psychiatry, it could be imagined that there is a large potential for MI also in psychiatric patients with alcohol or drug related disorders not meeting full criteria of a specific diagnosis. This is also supported by recently published data by Hansen et al. (2000), showing a significant under-diagnosing of substance related disorders in psychiatry. This is said to be followed by a lack of adequate treatment interventions. These facts could also mean that problems of efficacy of early intervention efforts are not only patient-related but also staff-related. In this context there have been reported several difficulties in implementing early intervention "packages" in general medical settings despite the fact that everybody strongly agreed that they are effective.

Competition of health care providers hinders financial support and clear responsibilities. Most effective treatment does not always translate into low costs for both purchasers and payers at first glance.

Today's clinical settings show a high grade of specialization with a great number of diagnostic and therapeutic tasks. It is therefore quite difficult to find a place for an additional intervention which does not necessarily deal with the actual primary task.

Lack of communication with specialized treatment facilities is one of the main problems and has already been discussed in the introduction section.

It has also been shown that there is a lack of skills in interviewing technique among medical professionals. Motivational interviewing techniques have to be learned by health professionals, because this specific interaction style is different from common medical counseling and advice.

Lack of support and supervision for the staff is often leading to resignative attitudes towards patients and „new methods" of intervention. Remarkably, it seems very destructive to the attitudes of the health professionals if a program was implemented but stopped after a while (Hamilton et al., 1994). In the field of substance related disorders, resignation among both patients and professionals can arise very quickly and lead to motivational depletion.

There is need for concrete measures to provide better implementation of early intervention or motivation enhancing interview techniques in the established health care system in the future.

First, enabling both purchasers and payers to provide financial support and leadership in the knowledge of long-term economic benefits of improved health among their clients.

Second, specific training for health professionals including workshops with skills training activities (role play, etc.). Inclusion of alcohol or drug related screening and intervention in quality improvement programs and financial gratifications or reimbursement of education time can also be used as vehicles for sustained implementation. Several books and manuals are available for training purposes (e.g. Miller and Rollnick, 2002; Connors et al., 2001).

Third, after the implementation of early intervention programs it is essential to provide sustained financial and professional support to the program and its protagonists. Thus, the implementation process has to include long-term perspectives.

Fourth, concrete steps can be taken to enhance the attention for substance related problems in medical fields like self-report tests, addition of specific questions to medical assessment routines, reminder systems, information booklets and contact possibilities with specialized institutions.

Fifth, it seems necessary to support the local proximity of primary health care and specialized therapy and to make patient related communication easier in terms of regular referral letters and clinical update exchange.

Which stage of change has been reached in modern health care systems concerning the prevention, awareness and active treatment of substance related disorders in "everyday health care life"? The rating will depend on the national health care developments in different countries, but overall it seems to be far from action or maintenance. Nevertheless, even precontemplation has its positive potentials.

References

Baker A, Lewin T, Reichler H, Clancy R, Carr V, Garrett R, Sly K, Devir H, Terry M (2002) Motivational interviewing among psychiatric in-patients with substance abuse disorders. Acta Psychiatr Scand 106(3): 233

Burke BL, Arkowitz H, Dunn C (2002) The efficacy of motivational interviewing and its adaptations. What we know so far. In: Miller WR, Rollnick S (eds) Motivational interviewing — preparing people for change, 2nd edn. Guilford Press, New York, p 237

Chick J (1991) Early intervention for hazardous drinking in the general hospital. Alc Alcohol [Suppl] 1: 477–479

Connors GJ, Donovan DM, DiClemente CC (2001) Substance abuse treatment and the stages of change. Guilford Press, London New York

DiClemente CC, Bellino LE, Neavins TM (1999) Motivation for change and alcoholism treatment. Alcohol Res Health 23(2): 86–92

Fleming MF, Baier Manwell L (1999) Brief intervention in primary care settings. A primary treatment method for at-risk, problem, and dependent drinkers. Alcohol Res Health 23(2): 128–137

Fleming MF, Barry KL, Manwell LB, Johnson K, London R (1997) Brief physician advice for problem alcohol drinkers. A randomized controlled trial in community-based primary care practices. JAMA 277(13): 1039–1045

Hamilton MR, Menkes DB, Jeffery AK (1994) Early intervention for alcohol misuse: encouraging doctors to take action. N Z Med J 107(989): 454–456

Handmaker N, Packard M, Conforti K (2002) Motivational interviewing in the treatment of dual disorders. In: Miller WR, Rollnick S (eds) Motivational interviewing — preparing people for change, 2nd edn. Guilford Press, New York, p 364

Hansen SS, Munk-Jørgensen P, Guldbæk T, Solgård T, Lauszus KS, Albrechtsen N, Borg L, Egander A, Faurholdt K, Gilberg A, Gosden NP, Lorenzen J, Richelsen B, Weischer K, Bertelsen A (2000) Psychoactive substance use diagnoses among psychiatric in-patients. Acta Psychiatr Scand 102(6): 432

Kristenson H, Ohlin H, Hulten-Nosslin MB, Trell E, Hood B (1983) Identification and intervention of heavy drinking in middle-aged men: results and follow-up of 24–60 months of long-term study with randomized controls. Alc Clin Exp Res 7(2): 203–209

Larimer ME, Kilmer JR (2000) Natural history. In: Zernig G, Saria A, Kurz M, O'Malley SS (eds) Handbook of alcoholism. CRC Press, Boca Raton London New York Washington, p 19

Miller WR, Rollnick S (eds) (2002) Motivational interviewing — preparing people for change, 2nd edn. Guilford Press, New York

Murray CJL, Lopez AD (1996) The global burden of disease: a comprehensive assessment of mortality and disability from diseases, injuries and risk factors in 1990 and projected. Harvard School of Public Health

Nilssen O (1991) The Tromso Study: identification of and a controlled intervention on a population of early-stage risk drinkers. Prev Med 20(4): 518–528

Prochaska JO, Norcross JC, DiClemente CC (1994) Changing for good. Harper Collins, New York

Regier DA, Farmer ME, Rae DS, Locks BZ, Keith SJ, Judd LL, Goodwin FK (1990) Comorbidity of mental disorders with alcohol and other drug abuse. JAMA 264: 2511–2518

Rice DP (1999) Economic costs of substance abuse, 1995. Proc Assoc Am Physicians 111(2): 119–125

Richmond R, Heather N, Wodak A, Kehoe L, Webster I (1995) Controlled evaluation of a general practice-based brief intervention for excessive drinking. Addiction 90(1): 119–132

Schwoon DR (1998) Motivierende Interventionen bei Suchtkranken. In: Gölz J (ed) Moderne Suchtmedizin. Diagnostik und Therapie der somatischen, psychischen und sozialen Syndrome. G Thieme, Stuttgart New York

Senft RA, Polen MR, Freedborn DK, Hollis JF (1997) Brief intervention in a primary care setting for hazardous drinkers. Am J Prev Med 13(6): 464–470

Sithartan T, Singh S, Kranitis P, Currie J, Freeman P, Murugesan G, Ludowicw J (1999) Aust NZ J Psychiatry 33: 676–635

Tomson Y, Romeslo A, Aberg H (1998) Excessive drinking — brief intervention by a primary health care nurse. A randomized controlled trial. Scand J Health Care 16(3): 188–192

Welte JW, Perry P, Longabaugh R, Clifford PR (1998) An outcome evaluation of a hospital-based early intervention program. Addiction 93(4): 573–581

Wienberg G (1995) Das Alkoholproblem in der medizinischen Primärversorgung. In: Mann K, Buchkremer G (eds) Suchtforschung und Suchttherapie in Deutschland. Sucht Sonderband, p 13

WHO Brief Intervention Study Group (1996) A cross-national trial of brief interventions with heavy drinkers. Am J Public Health 86(7): 948–955

Author's address: M. Kurz, MD, Assoc. Prof., Therapie und Gesundheitszentrum Mutters, Innsbruck University Hospital, Department of Psychiatry, Nockhofweg 23, A-6162 Mutters, Austria, e-mail: martin.kurz@uklibk.ac.at

Homogenizing alcoholism treatment across Europe

F. Poldrugo

Department of Mental Health, University of Trieste, Italy

Summary. Alcohol treatment ideologies and goals vary in different countries of Europe and have been influenced by cultures and drinking patterns. From the traditional high-consumption wine countries of Southern Europe to the spirit drinking North European countries. However, due to the natural course of alcoholism, long-term alcohol dependent patients share common features independent from initial drinking patterns and cultural influences. This makes populations' characteristics and the result of treatment comparable within Europe, even though treatment approaches and selection of patients vary in different countries. Clinical trials using common measures for outcome of intervention have been performed in the last ten years in several countries of Europe. Outcome has been measured not only with the traditional definition of abstinence (or other drinking end-points), but also in terms of the subjective impact of disease and treatments on patients' lives. The discovery that different types of supportive therapies (alone or in combination with medications) do have positive influences on the progress of the alcoholic disease, improving the patients' quality of life (QoL) in all countries of Europe, shed a light of optimism on what, until recently, was considered an untreatable disease.

Summary — From the age when alcohol treatment outcomes were incorrectly measured and barely comparable because of different populations (especially from the USA), scarce description of intervention and goals of treatment, a great progress has been reached, in recent years, with new methodologies applied in Europe in clinical trials dealing with populations of alcoholics. Therapies do work in improving their well-being status and life expectancy in all countries of Europe.

Introduction

The European Community is becoming a reality pushing countries with different histories and customs to co-exist and integrate. However, this will be a very long process since diversities are paramount at present. The field of alcohol use and alcoholism is not immune from these diversities. Different drinking patterns exist because of different attitudes, values, and perceptual constructs. Different legal and health systems also funnel different kind of clients to alcohol treatment systems. The goals of treatment may also differ. We are dealing with a complex situation with a minimal support from the literature since the field of alcohol treatment is relatively new. We shall start by describing differences using criteria to compare the existing treatments, and focusing on the discovery of common features useful for treatment all over Europe.

The health systems in Europe

Even a scanty description and comparison of the health systems at work in the various regions of Europe does not exist. It would be simplistic to think that the same standard of cure is offered to all European citizens. As an example, a recent research considering the number, education, way of practice, relationship with specialist alcohol treatment centers, and reimbursement mechanisms of General Practitioners (GPs) throughout Europe (with the aim to understand the existing potentialities in early detection and intervention on subjects with alcoholic problems) demonstates great diversities (Walburg, 2001). Existing health policies differ, even though, in Europe, most of the programs for alcoholics are provided by the public services. In the USA, instead, the health system operates through the private and public market and alcoholics are inevitably selected for treatment on the basis of their economic resources (and type of insurance coverage). Also the philosophy underlying public intervention varies among different countries, thus directing different types of alcoholics to different treatment facilities. For example, legislation may be limited to either alcohol problems (e.g. Hungary), or drug problems (in Italy a law considering alcohol and alcohol-related problems is in force only since April 2001); or both either separately (e.g. Sweden) or combined (e.g. Finland). Alternatively, addiction may be covered by mental health acts (e.g. UK). Some countries consider also compulsory treatment, but the grounds for intervention vary from the need of caring for the alcoholic's family (e.g. Switzerland), to the need of curing alcohol-related ailments (e.g. with special reference to mental health in the UK), or to control public order (e.g. Finland) and social conformity (e.g. legislation in former Soviet Union) (Havard, 1992).

Drinking patterns in Europe

Cultural, racial, and religious traditions are linked to variations in patterns of alcohol use. The Mediterranean area, since the Greek and Roman times, has been a major region for the production and consumption of wine; wine continues to be the principal beverage. In Italy wine is symbolically related to the blood of Christ in the celebration of the mass. This linking of blood and wine has led to an elaborate health belief system closely associating wine with food, nourishment, good digestion, strength for hard work, good blood, and generally well-being and good health. Wine is consumed for its social and presumed nutritional value instead of its psychological effects. It is consumed daily (in moderation), usually around mealtimes by the whole family, including young children. Drunkenness is frowned upon and is relatively uncommon. Although, to a certain extent, the French mimic the Italian practice of drinking wine with meals, the French have traditionally experienced higher rates of drinking problems. In both countries, wine is consumed copiously by the entire population, and children are initiated early into the drinking customs. There the similarity stops. The French experience a high incidence of drunkenness and alcoholism; the rates of death from alcoholism and cirrhosis of the liver in France has been among the highest in the world. This may be related to differences in attitudes. In Italy, drunkenness is socially unacceptable; in France, intoxication is viewed as a sign of manhood, and there is a wide tolerance on copious drinking.

Traditional attitudes toward alcohol use in peasant Poland as in other Eastern European countries (e.g. former Yugoslavia, Soviet Union, etc.) treated it as a necessary part of socializing and a symbol of hospitality. Alcohol is used for a variety of purposes including sealing contracts, marking life events, and celebrating. Drinking occurs after, rather than during, meals. The drink of choice is distilled spirits, typically vodka or whiskey. Drinking is primarily a male activity, and alcohol is associated with virility and manhood; both heavy drinking and drunkenness are tolerated. Sanctions only occur when drinking result in the neglect of the individual's moral duties toward family and church.

Drinking in the Scandinavian countries, as in Poland, is characterized by the separation of drinking from dietary functions, a preference for distilled spirits, the deliberate use of alcohol to produce intoxication, and the concentration of heavy drinking in a relatively small portion of the male population.

In England, Scotland, Ireland drinking patterns are similar. However, Protestant churches (as the Baptists, Presbyterians, and Congregationalists) exerted a strong influence on drinking strongly opposing alcohol use and viewing drunkenness as sinful, and, later on, influencing the temperance movement. But attaining male identity is intimately bound to the ethic of hard drinking of all these countries. Later on drinking became even a symbol of Irish identity.

In Germany, permissive attitudes toward drinking and drunkenness persist today. There are preferences for wine in the wine-growing regions, for spirits in former East Germany, and for beer in Bavaria; however, beer is the first choice of frequent and regular drinkers. In Switzerland different types of drinking patterns exist considering its Italian, French and German speaking areas.

A special case is the traditional Orthodox Jewish community which is scattered in all countries of Europe. Here alcoholic beverages, particularly wine, have a symbolic role in religious celebrations associated with rites of passage, weekly Sabbath observances, and annual holy days and festivals. Unlike other cultures in which festivals are seen as times for pleasure seeking and convivial drinking, true rejoicing and festivity are integral with worship and contingent on conformity with religious customs and fulfillment of ritual obligations. It follows that in the Jewish culture, Jews do not drink with the aim of getting drunk or feeling good. Drinking is not sought for its psychological effects. Rather, Jews develop a ritual attitude toward drinking in which drinking for the effect of alcohol is alien to them. As a result, although few Jews abstain from alcohol, the rate of alcoholism among Jews is lower than in any other cultural group.

Diversities of drinking patterns lead also to recognition of the necessity of culturally informed strategies of intervention. This is not a peregrine idea since some existing widespread communities (like the Jews present in all Europe) have peculiar necessities, but, especially, for the great mobility of citizens belonging to different cultures within the European community. It has also to be recognized that some cultures (like the Spanish, Italian and Portuguese which are family centered) are most successful not only in preventing alcohol abuse but also in treating alcohol diseases (Sanchez Sosa and Poldrugo, 2001). The members of such cultures tend to: 1) view alcohol as a natural, normal part of life about which they have no ambivalence; 2) teach their young by example how to drink in moderation; 3) encourage drinking among family and friends rather than in same-gender settings; 4) discourage heavy episodic drinking; 5) sanction negatively and promptly any unacceptable drinking behavior; 6) respect the decision of those who choose not to drink and not pressure them to drink; 7) be free of the belief that alcohol can solve problems, signify adulthood, grant power, or confirm manhood (Hanson, 1995).

The alcohol treatment systems

As a rule of thumb countries characterized by "binge drinking" (e.g. Finland, Sweden and UK) have more treatment facilities, since it has been demonstrated that the number of treatment programs reflects the extension of behavioral consequences of drinking and the proportion of beverages consumed as spirits (Takala et al., 1992). By contrast, countries where wine consumption is integrated in dietary habits (like Italy and France), even if alcohol (wine) consumption is greater, have fewer treatment facilities. In the Mediterranean countries of Europe, spontaneous remission is rare, and alcoholics are treated in medical wards because of the prominent physical disturbances (e.g. liver cirrhosis, GI tract diseases, pancreatitis, etc.).

It is true that differences between countries in both beverage choices and alcohol-consumption levels have been diminishing. However, the trend toward homogenization is far from complete.

The management of alcohol-related problems could be divided into four components where 1) the manipulation of drinking patterns and levels of intake is only part of it, and the other 2) the control of disruptive behavior, 3) the provision of material services and spiritual confort to needy or unhappy drinkers, and 4) treatment of alcohol-related medical complications may combine, and there are often ambiguous gliding from one component to the other.

Uncontroversially, "treatment" applies only to alcohol-related medical complications and this will be the main focus of this chapter even though medical treatment could not be consider in a vacuum like in the "black-box" evaluation paradigm (Moos et al., 1990).

Treatment is markedly influenced by the life stressors, spiritual needs as well as by the cultural and social context (which are contextually included in the definition of QoL).

The life-course view of dependence

Subjects achieving abstinence show varying outcomes depending on sample characteristics, outcome definition, and completeness of follow-up. Most but not all reports describe an intermediate category of "social" or "asymptomatic" drinking lying between abstinence and continued problematic drinking. These subjects are probably a mix of patients who were never severely dependent, those who were sliding toward relapse, and those drinking with lowered tolerance to alcohol.

Valuable insights in the understanding of the multidetermined nature of alcoholism have come from follow-up studies on cohorts of subjects recruited not for their drinking but for some other purpose, but with the ensuing drinking behavior then prospectively explored. Vaillant (1983) acknowledged that besides multidetermined causes, alcoholism, once developed, is chronic. In the III stage of drinking progress, about 3 per cent to 5 per cent of American adults (men outnumber women 3 or 4 to 1) become physical dependent on alcohol. Once addiction has occurred, the individual progresses to social incapacity or death. Spontaneous recovery is generally uncommon. Sobriety may be reached by detoxification and treatment, including the use of support groups.

This is also the case for the clinical populations throughout Europe where most of the subjects are severely dependent with 3–4 fold excess mortality compared with age-matched controls (Poldrugo et al., 1993). The toll of years lost in alcoholics is very high. With the progression of the disease and the expression of its biological nature, symptoms become less dependent on drinking patterns, and on social and environmental factors. Alcoholics die about 20 years earlier than expected. A mean age of death at 50–55 years has been reported in most countries, independent of the geographical area considered (e.g. Europe, USA or Japan) (Poldrugo, 1999a) (Table 1).

Among 100 patients treated for alcohol dependence who were aged 45 years at the intake point and followed for 20 years, about 40% would have died by the 20-year anniversary. Of the remaining subjects over 30% will still be experiencing continued or intermittent trouble with their drinking and rather less than 30% will be abstinent or engaging in trouble-free drinking. Recovery from drinking problems is generally, but not necessarily, associated with consequent improvement in health, social functioning and QoL (Poldrugo, 2001).

Table 1. Mortality rates in different populations of alcoholics

Population Mortality	Country	Interval (years)	Sample size	No. of deaths	(%)
Community samples					
Thorarinsson	Iceland	±13	2,863	573	20
Ojesjo	Sweden	15	96	25	26
Alcohol treatment facilities					
Norvig and Nielsen	Denmark	4	221	42	19
Lundquist	Sweden	9	200	46	23
Verbanck et al.	Belgium	10	121	29	24
Psychiatric populations					
Lesch et al.	Austria	±5	444	101	23
Poldrugo and Fiore	Italy	5	995	231	23
Lindelius et al.	Sweden	5–10	257	44	17
Nicholls et al.	UK	10–15	935	309	33
Berglund	Sweden	±18	1,312	537	41
O'Connor et al.	UK	20	133	53	40

Evaluation of treatment of alcohol dependence

In recent years European Guidelines for alcohol treatment appeared following the already existing American and Canadian ones (The Plinius Maior Society, 1994). This came out of the need to perform clinical trials for alcohol treatment with the same standards used with other drugs to treat other chronic diseases. Today drugs specific to alcohol treatment are available. This has an enormous impact on the alcohol field since, as for other psychiatric diseases, the availability of drug therapy helps to abate resistance in intervening on apparently untreatable diseases.

To address alcohol treatment three dimensions should be considered: a) patient description; b) intervention description; and c) outcome measurements. Of course, all the instruments used to classify and compare should be translated and validated cross-culturally. This is an uneasy task since instruments are frequently distributed in limited cultural circuits (e.g. Latin, Scandinavian countries, etc.), or resent of the prevailing Anglo-Saxon scientific culture. International agencies coordinating cross-cultural efforts had limited impact so far although the ongoing reorganization of European agencies will bring, in the near future, a major contribution in the field.

Patient and population description

The description of the patient and of clinical signs is typical of the medical approach. The CAGE questionnaire has been widely in use for very brief screening but is oversensitive in the "drier" countries of Northern Europe and misses many dependent drinkers in Southern Europe where there is less guilt and concern about alcohol. In medical setting the Alcohol Use Disorders

Identification Test (AUDIT) is advisable having being validated in a number of countries. Several official internationally recognized diagnostic criteria exist. A very useful criteria to compare is the Addiction Severity Index (ASI) which has been validated also at the European level. These instruments include description of drinking patterns too.

Psychiatric problems associated with alcohol misuse should also be considered. Primary and secondary alcoholism may have different prognosis. The use of the Diagnostic and Statistical Manual of Mental Disorders (Revised) (DSM-III and IV) is standard current practice in Europe. The social environment can also be measured with the previous questionnaires. For international comparative research purposes the Symptom Check List (Revised) (SCL-90-R) is the only easy to use symptom inventory available that provides sufficient coverage of important areas of psychopathological symptomatology.

QoL is another variable to be considered in alcoholics entering treatment programs. The Short Form (SF-36) Health Survey Questionnaire, though designed for the use in outcomes studies in general medical patients, is seen as relevant by alcohol dependent subjects. For this reason the test can be used to compare handicap between different diseases, and to help prioritize the distribution of healthcare resources. It is quick to complete, and gives a score for physical and social functioning, role limitation, physical and mental well-being and an overall health perception and health change. It has been translated in different languages. The Mental Health Division of the World Health Organization (WHO) is also developing a similar instrument for cross-cultural use. Other instruments measuring cognitive functions, motivation to treatment and spirituality have been recently developed but yet not cross-validated in Europe.

Biological tests for chronic excessive consumption should be barely influenced by life and social context. But there is a need for standardization of methodologies across Europe in relation to multinational cooperative research and treatment programs.

Transaminases, gamma-glutamyl transferase (GGT), the mean (cell) corpuscular volume (MCV) are included in ordinary blood tests, and carbohydrate-deficient transferrin (CDT), which is a prominent marker for continuous heavy alcohol consumption with a high degree of specificity is now available all over Europe (Poldrugo and Allen, 1999).

Today, also in the alcohol field, information drawn for any single patient may be used in epidemiological studies considering entire populations. Data on alcohol use, severity of alcoholism, and QoL allow us to have an idea of similarities and differences existing before treatments start among clinical populations of different European countries. Data on mortality are also highly valuable to describe characteristics and needs of large populations, as well as treatment outcome, with the aim to compare data from different countries (Poldrugo, 1999a; Poldrugo et al., 1993). Database which are property of insurance companies could be useful as well, both in the general and clinical populations, but are not yet available to alcohol researchers in Europe (Holder and Blose, 1992).

Intervention description

Therapeutic approaches involve different psychotherapies (behavioral, cognitive, psychodynamic), sociotherapy, support therapies (like those provided by the Alcoholics Anonymous -AA, and the Clubs for Treated Alcoholics — CATs, mutual-help groups or similar associations), and medications. This variety does not ease the collection of comparable data; moreover interventions are normally mixed. Description of treatment is rarely rigorous. For some psychotherapies, only recently reference manuals have appeared but not as yet in Europe.

GPs are the key contact figures early on in the intervention for addictive disorders (Poldrugo, 1999b). They see 71% of the general population every year, but their capacity for detecting alcoholism is very low. There are different reasons for their reluctance to initiate treatment, among which previous negative experience with treatment outcome and their own personal drinking. Although minimal intervention programs are encouraged, GPs refer to specialized agencies both problem drinkers and alcohol-dependent patients. About 90% of clients do not comply with the referral suggestions and thus miss treatment options.

Treatment settings may vary. Besides primary care, programs may be organized at the work site, by the criminal justice system (treatment as an alternative to sentencing; treatment imposed by courts; treatment in prison; treatment for drink-driving offenders), by community alcohol teams but, in the everyday world, most alcoholics are referred to hospitals. Specialist alcohol treatment centers in general funnel, among alcohol dependent subjects, those more "vulnerable" to physical and mental effects of alcohol or those patients that "mature out of dependence".

Detoxification, in Europe, still plays a major part in the initiation of the treatment of alcohol addicts. It is seldom conducted alone but usually integrated by external support (either general psychological or specific physchoterapies). The most common procedure is inpatient detoxification conducted in psychiatric and general hospitals (comprising university clinics), seldom in private clinics, with a stay no longer than 14 days. Inpatient rehabilitation in residential settings (for a maximum stay of 3 months) and long-term rehabilitation, performed on an outpatient basis, is provided in most countries. It is commonly agreed that attendance to mutual-help groups becomes a part of a wider long-term rehabilitation program. Here, the different arrangements for providing healthcare in the countries of Europe are coming to play; some approaches are more or less popular depending to culture. In many countries there is a combination of provision by the state, by private organizations, and by voluntary organizations or charities. The Salvation Army programs are typical of the UK and Scandinavia. In the Mediterranean countries, where social pressure is the major determinant of relapse, and where citizens are fully covered by public health plans, sociotherapy is integrated within programs that are organized at the community level. The system of the Clubs was expanded in former Yugoslavia. Similar programs are at present successfully applied in different cultural contexts. The Clubs are present in the

Table 2. Treatment differences between the Clubs for Treated Alcoholics (CATs) and Alcoholic Anonymous (AA) Groups

Clubs of Treated Alcoholics	Alcoholic Anonymous
Addiction as a family style	addiction as an illness
Alcoholics and families	independent family groups
Change in lifestyle	12 steps
Social functions	no social functions
Visibility in the community	anonymity
Complex associative structure	no associative structure
± relationship with the medical system	independent from the medical system
± use of drugs (e.g. disulfiram)	no medications
Trained therapists	no therapists

Eastern European countries (Croatia, Slovenia, Poland, Serbia, and more recently in Russia and Moldovia), Italy, Spain, Portugal, Scandinavia (e.g. in Denmark), South America (Chile) and Oceania (New Zealand). The AA groups, instead, follow a philosophy related to the search of spiritual values which are universal and less related to culture. They are present all over Europe. The differences in philosophies of treatment relevant to the two most important mutual-help associations of Europe are seen on Table 2 (Poldrugo, 1997).

Several professional roles contribute to therapy in the field: medical doctors, nurses, social workers, occupational therapists, psychologists, counselors, and psychotherapists. What is fundamental is to organize interactions as a teamwork, and co-operation between organization giving provisions.

Outpatient treatment, a more intense intervention, a longer stay in treatment, and the stability of the treatment environment seem to play a major role in treatment of alcohol dependent subjects, but the key issue is participation of patients in aftercare.

Outcome measurements

Following an alcohol dependent patient during treatment means participation in a continuous process of change influencing the results. Intensive experimental follow-up will bring better results which unfortunately cannot be applied to a naturalistic setting. The goals of treatment will dictate the primary outcome measures. They must not be too ambitious to avoid relapse due to unrealistic expectations. Recovery from severe alcohol dependence almost inevitably involves personal acceptance of an abstinence goal. For this reason still the most used outcome measures relate to abstinence and drinking behaviors with its variations of cumulative abstinence duration (CAD), time to first drink, or interval between the first drink and relapse. More than with other illnesses, the process of follow-up is combined with compliance, and good compliance is predictive and equivalent to a good outcome. Other outcome measures may consist of returning to normal values of biological markers. Improvement in clinical status, severity of addiction, psychological and mental measurements, and social functioning are other outcomes under consideration. An improvement in family's health and well-being is a very important goal, since problems affecting spouse and children are of wide proportions and expensive to society. A global outcome, combining different outcome dimensions, is considered by the instruments measuring variations from initial baseline of QoL of alcoholic patients. A global, and objective measurement, to be used in a naturalistic setting, minimizing loss at follow-up, which is sensitive to intervention, is the study of mortality rates in larger populations (Poldrugo, 1999a).

In recent years some meta-analysis have appeared about treatment that apparently work (Holder et al., 1991; Finney and Monahan, 1996). For the aforementioned methodological discussions on differences between treatments and goals of treatment this approach leads to an oversimplification of the result, but is still a valuable critical approach.

Evaluating alcohol treatment outcome across Europe

The primary treatment for alcohol dependence is psycho-social support and counseling, with drug treatment mostly being considered as adjuvant or secondary. Drug trial design should hence consider the measurement of the adjuvant drug effect, while at the same time assuring equal principal therapy. However, as discussed above, due to differences in individual patient psychosocial profiles and variation in psychoterapeutic methodology, centers, cultures and countries, the standardization of equal principal therapy to all patients may be a methodological obstacle. However, the large scale use of acamprosate throughout Europe has provided a unique opportunity to compare the treatments existing in different countries of Europe and their outcome. A number of phase II, III and IV studies have been conducted on more than 4000 patients in various European countries including the UK, Belgium, The Netherlands, Switzerland, Germany, Austria, France, Italy and Portugal (Sojka, 1996). This is the largest database existing in the world assuring sufficient sample size to contrast high variability and the expected modest success rates, whichever treatment is used. The usefulness of this database derives from the fact that all studies followed a core protocol and were carried out in accordance with the guidelines of good clinical practice in Europe. Trials lasted 6–12 months in order to take into account the addictive and chronic nature of the disease, the natural tendencies for fluctuation of drinking patterns and motivation, and the major influence of social and life events on behavior and coping mechanisms. The primary outcome criteria were: abstinence/relapse/missing assessment at each visit, time to first relapse, CAD. Substantial effort was taken to measure alcohol intake adequately and to obtain any possible information on patients who dropped out during the treatment phase or follow-up. The information base included detailed interviews and information from GPs and family members. Biological markers

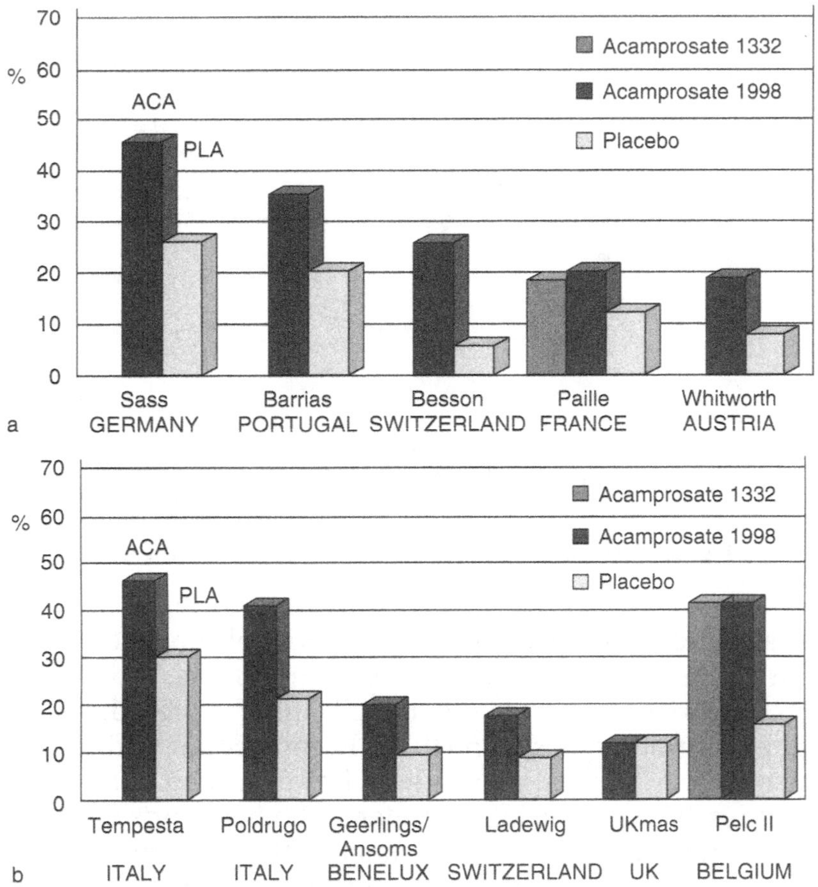

Fig. 1. Survival analysis comparing acamprosate (ACA) and placebo (PLA). **a** Studies with 12-month (48-week) treatment phase. **b** Studies with 3- or 6-month treatment phase

were measured in all studies. Thus the obtained data for abstinence/relapse may be consider valid. With the exception of the study conducted in the UK all clinical trials clearly indicated acamprosate to be superior to placebo with respect to abstinence rate in various clinical settings and countries of Europe (Fig. 1). Interestingly, rates of abstinence in controls were higher in community-based alcohol rehabilitation programs like in those of Germany, Portugal and Italy; the biological impact of the drug was more marked, instead, in programs using individual therapies like those of the Switzerland and The Netherlands. The same results have been confirmed lately in a study which also included data from Spain and Sweden (Potgieter and Lehert, 1999). As the study complied with the Cochrane A requirements, this enhanced the generalisibility of the data.

More recently, acamprosate has been used in the New European Alcoholism Treatment (NEAT) program which is an open-label multicenter clinical trial conducted in 6 European countries (Fuchs, 1999). Data from 5 countries are available. The objective of the study, beside assessing the efficacy of the drug, was to asses patient profiles and QoL. Patients recruited were 1,258. In

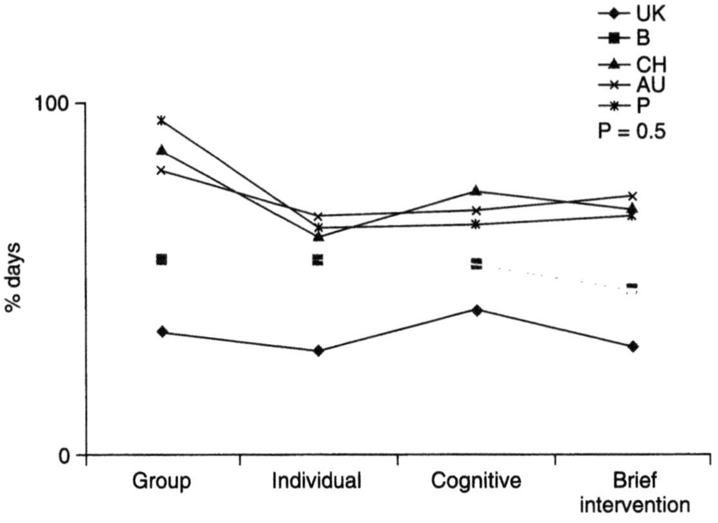

Fig. 2. Percent days non-relapse by psychosocial report

these clinical populations age of onset and severity of dependence were similar in all countries. DSM-III mean scores were: 7.2 in Austria, 7.0 in Belgium, 7.3 in Portugal, 6.8 in Switzerland and 8.0 in the UK. Interestingly drinking at home, free of cultural attributes, was found to be the most common drinking environment in all countries. Clinical populations, however, were differently selected across countries. The proportion of patient who had a prison history ranged from 6% in Belgium to 32% in the UK; similarly the proportion of patients who declared that they were unemployed as a result of their alcohol dependence was lowest in Belgium (16%) and highest in the UK (43%). After the alcohol-related health complicances, family influences were the primary reason for seeking treatment in all countries demonstrating that, for alcohol dependent subjects, excessive alcohol consumption is often, and incorrectly, considered a private problem (Orford, 1994). Preferences for psychotherapies varied between countries. Individual psychotherapy was the most common method requested in Switzerland (63%), cognitive behavioral therapy (CBT) was preferred in the UK (54%), and group therapy was requested most in Austria (40%) and Portugal (54%). There was a trend toward an improved outcome with group therapy (Fig. 2). The number of patient discontinuations ranged from 38–41% in Austria, Portugal and Switzerland to 80% in the UK. There was a marked reduction in alcohol consumption in patients who relapse. In all countries the majority of compliant patients were abstinent at last assessment. QoL improved after treatment with a fairly strong connection with abstinence and compliance (Poldrugo and Lehert, 2001) (Fig. 3).

Conclusions

Even though the field of alcoholism is relatively new, clarification of treatment goals, and refined methodological approaches for assessment of drinking

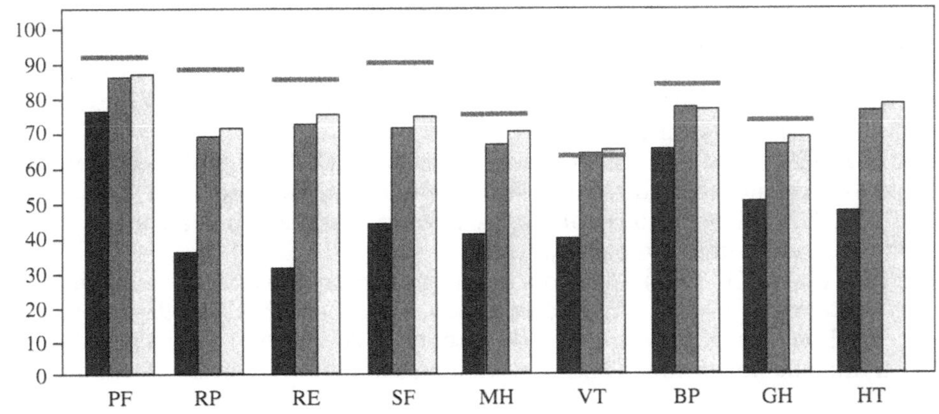

Fig. 3. Evolution of scores on the different dimensions of the SF 36 during the NEAT study. *PF* physical functioning, *RP* role limitations due to physical problems, *RE* role limitations due to emotional problems, *SF* social functioning, *MH* mental health, *VT* energy and vitality, *BP* bodily pain, *GH* general health perception, *HT* health transition over time. Data are presented as the mean ± SEM of values obtained from the compliant patients that reached the time-point. ■ represent data at baseline (n = 1,258), ■ those at 3 months (n = 720) and ▨ those at 6 months (n = 511). The solid horizontal red lines correspond to values from the reference population (Jenkinson et al., 1993)

behavior and the clinical status during treatment intervention, have contributed to grant a scientific background to this medical field. Standardization of criteria on evaluation of treatment of alcohol dependence at European level (The Plinius Maior Society, 1994) and the discovery that alcoholics in the long term are less affected by cultural attributes (Poldrugo, 1999a) have given a new insight into treatment of alcoholism with commonalties found throughout Europe and a possibility of comparison with the rest of the world.

We now are aware that alcohol treatment does work in all countries, that different outcomes are expected based on different types of intervention, that a drug adjuvant to treatments already available increase positive treatment outcomes. Since alcoholism, among chronic diseases, has the peculiar capacity to disrupt the alcoholic's social context (Berkman and Syme, 1979), recent studies, conducted in several countries of Europe, have paid more attention to factors outside treatment that are the primary determinant of remission and relapses, such as stressful life circumstances, and the lack of social resources. Treatment compliance and the establishment of new relationships in a non-drinking network, more than changes in civil status and working situation, were equivalent to abstinence in improving QoL in alcoholics.

References

Berkman LF, Syme SL (1979) Social network, social resistance, and mortality: a nine-year follow-up of Alameda County residents. Am J Epidemiol 109: 186–204

Finney JW, Monahan SC (1996) The cost-effectiveness of treatment for alcoholism: a second approximation. J Stud Alcohol 57: 229–243
Fuchs WJ (1999) The European NEAT programme. In: The added value of acamprosate in clinical practice. Proceedings, ESBRA Satellite Symposium. Barcelona, 1999. Adis, Oxford (Drugs in Focus, pp 13–15)
Hanson DJ (1995) The United States of America. In: Heath DW (ed) International handbook on alcohol and culture. Greenwood Press, Westport, CT
Havard D (1992) Alcohol abuse and legislation in Europe. In: L'alcologia in Europa. Editrice Compositori, Bologna, pp 1–12
Holder HD, Blose JO (1992) The reduction of health care costs associated with alcoholism treatment: a 14-year longitudinal study. J Stud Alcohol 53: 293–302
Holder H, Longabaugh R, Miller WR, Rubonis AV (1991) The cost-effectiveness of treatment for alcoholism: a first approximation. J Stud Alcohol 52: 517–540
Jenkinson C, Coulter A, Wright L (1993) Short Form 36 (SF36) Health Survey Questionnaire: normative data for adults of working age. Br Med J 306: 1437–1440
Moos RH, Finney JW, Cronkite RC (1990) Alcoholism treatment. Context, process and outcome. Oxford University Press, New York London
Orford J (1994) Empowering families and friends: a new approach to secondary prevention of addiction. Drug Alcohol Rev 13: 417–430
The Plinius Maior Society (1994) Guidelines on evaluation of treatment of alcohol dependence. Alcoholism: J Alcohol Alcohol-related Dis 30 [Suppl 1]: 1–83
Poldrugo F (1997) Integration of pharmacotherapies in the existing programs for the treatment of alcoholics: an international perspective. In: Miller N (ed) The integration of pharmacological and nonpharmacological treatments in drug/alcohol addictions. The Haworth Medical Press, Binghamton, NY, pp 65–82
Poldrugo F (1999a) Mortality studies in the long-term evaluation of treatment of alcoholics. Alcoscope 2(2): 4–6
Poldrugo F (1999b) Recognition and treatment of alcohol-related disorders in primary care. Alcoscope 2(4): 12–15
Poldrugo F (2001) Quality of life and alcohol dependence. Alcoscope 4(2): 12–12
Poldrugo F, Allen J (1999) Biochemical markers of alcohol problems. ICAA Monograph, Lausanne, pp 1–59
Poldrugo F, Lehert P (2002) Acamprosate and quality of life. In: Progress in alcoholism management. Proceedings Symposium, Trieste 2001. Adis, Oxford (Drug Ther Perspect 1: 19–24)
Poldrugo F, Urizzi R (1993) The Italian Paradox: treatment initiatives and falling alcohol consumption. In: Klingemann H, Takala JP, Hunt G (eds) Care, cure or control. Alcoholism treatment in sixteen countries. State University of New York Press, Albany, NY, pp 191–204
Poldrugo F, Chick J, Moore N, Walburg A (1993) Mortality studies in the long-term evaluation of treatment of alcoholics. Alcohol Alcoholism 28 [Suppl 2]: 151–155
Potgieter AS, Lehert P (1999) Pooled analysis of the European study programme. In: The added value of acamprosate in clinical practice. Proceedings, ESBRA Satellite Symposium. Barcelona, 1999. Adis, Oxford (Drugs in Focus, pp 10–12)
Sanchez-Sosa JJ, Poldrugo F (2001) The role of the family. In: Houghton E, Roche AM (eds) Brunner/Routledge, Philadelphia, PA, pp 57–83
Sojka M (1996) Clinical efficacy of acamprosate in the treatment of alcoholism. In: Soyka M (ed) Acamprosate in relapse prevention of alcoholism. Springer, Berlin Heidelberg New York Tokyo, pp 155–171
Takala JP, Klingemann H, Hunt G (1992) Afterword: common directions and remaining divergences. In: Klingemann H, Takala JP, Hunt G (eds) Care, cure or control. Alcoholism treatment in sixteen countries. State University of New York Press, Albany, NY, pp 285–304

Vaillant G (1983) The natural history of alcoholism. Harvard University Press, Cambridge, MA
Walburg (2001) personal communication

Author's address: F. Poldrugo, MD, Ph.D., Office for Research and Innovative Projects on Alcohol, other Addictions and Mental Health, Departments of Mental Health and Addictions, University of Trieste/School of Medicine and The Community Health Agency, Piazzale Luigi Canestrini, 4, I-34126 Trieste, Italy, e-mail: polydrug@units.it

Springer-Verlag and the Environment